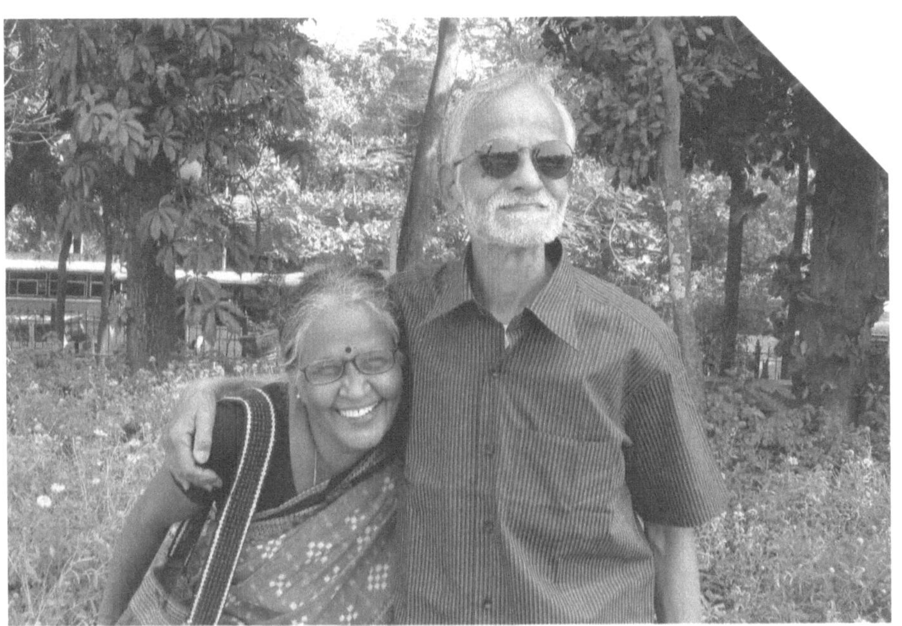

> **To dad and mom.
> This book is a convergence
> of everything I ever learnt
> from you. It is proof
> of my growing up,
> my gratitude and
> my deep love for you.**

I dedicate this book to my parents. For them health was always the ultimate wealth. They tried to teach me this while I was young. I didn't listen. Today I understand its infinite value and wish that I had acknowledged and lived their advice from the word Go.

DEVELOP YOUR DIABETES QUOTIENT

WRITTEN SPECIALLY FOR

THE TYPE 2 INDIAN DIABETIC!

GEETA AIYER
A TYPE 2 DIABETIC
SINCE 2006
**CERTIFIED DIABETES
EDUCATOR** (NDEP)

CHAPTER 9:
THE ULTIMATE SHORT-CUT TO DIABETES MANAGEMENT.

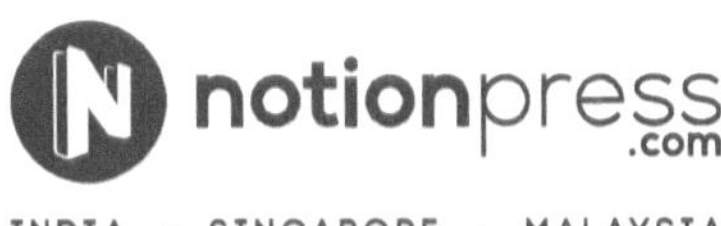

INDIA • SINGAPORE • MALAYSIA

Notion Press

No.8, 3rd Cross Street
CIT Colony, Mylapore
Chennai, Tamil Nadu – 600004

First Published by Notion Press 2021
Copyright © Geeta Aiyer 2021
All Rights Reserved.

ISBN 978-1-63873-564-9

FOREWORD

Foreword by Dr. Rajendra Thorat

"As a Diabetologist I see a variety of patients every single day. Whenever a new diabetic comes to me, I spend at least 30-60 minutes with that patient to explain the basics of diabetes and what an unmanaged and untreated diabetes can lead to. It is then for individual patients to comply through lifestyle changes along with the treatment plan that I propose for them."

"But diabetes is an on-going condition and the initial motivation to do well and maintain healthy sugar levels may sometimes take a backseat as life takes over. While there is always the intent to justify and maximise a patient's time with me, it does become impractical due to time and other constraints. This is where 'Develop Your Diabetes Quotient' steps in. For a type 2 diabetic, this book is a must-have, as it acts as a constant source of reminder through its unique approach to diabetes management - experiential and practical backed by medically sound information. This book excellently combines a patient's perspective and a diabetes educator's point-of-view."

"I congratulate Geeta on being able to narrate her diabetes-related experiences so well and put it all together for the benefit of type 2 diabetics all over India and across the globe. My very best to her and to 'Develop Your Diabetes Quotient'."

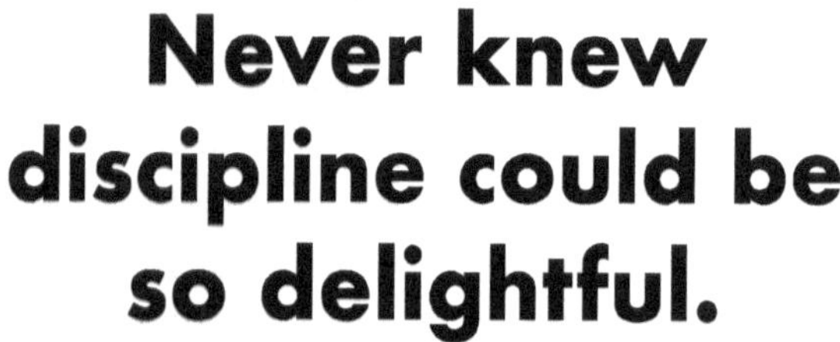

Never knew discipline could be so delightful.

- Geeta Aiyer

Co-Founder - The unDiplomatic Diabetic

INTRODUCTION

Diabetes is a multifaceted, back-breaking climb that manifests itself physically, mentally, emotionally, socially, financially and professionally. In each living moment, every diabetic is waging an uphill battle. Whether you are a newly diagnosed diabetic or someone already living with it, you would have realised that this condition is an expedition with only a beginning. There is no end in sight, yet.

Over the 14 odd years of being a type 2 diabetic, I have lived through the worst phases of this condition and today probably living its best. I was obsessed with getting better and during that journey my mind accumulated very many facts, figures, shades and nuances of this condition. All this resulted in reaching a benign HbA1c of 5.8 (average blood sugar level of 120) from a difficult and dangerous 10 (average blood sugar level of 240). Collectively, these experiences gave me what I call my 'Diabetes Quotient'. 'Diabetes Quotient' is 'parallel intelligence'. It is something only a diabetic can attempt to have. And once you develop it, it can become your best friend and your biggest asset.

'Develop Your Diabetes Quotient' is a bower, a pit-stop, a base-camp, an oasis - call it what you like. What it aims to do is single-mindedly help every diabetic revive, restore and rejuvenate for the next phase of their diabetic life.

I have written this book as
a diabetic patient who is averaging
an HbA1c of 6 for the last 5 years.
My best HbA1c in this tenure has
been 5.8 and I haven't gone
beyond 6.6. I have also written
this book as a certified diabetes
educator. This book aims to
complement the advice given
by your doctor. It does not
in any which way replace your
doctor's advice.

Further, this book has been
validated for medical correctness
by Dr. Rajendra Thorat -
(M.B.B.S., M.D. (MUM), PGDDM
Middlesex University (U.K.),
PGDHSc, Dip. (Diabetology),
Fellowship In Diabetology, CCGDM,
CCEBDM, International Diabetes
Federation Recognised).

I thank Dr. Thorat for his valuable
time and inputs in making this book
as close to perfect as it can be.

CHAPTERS

IT NEVER WAS YOUR FAULT...

IT NEVER WAS YOUR FAULT...

01 ▶ **... but you sure were a catalyst**

As you begin to read this book, let me assure you that **10 out of the 12 chapters in this book are solution-oriented.** They offer you a way of revisiting and relooking at your own or your loved one's diabetes management. They address lifestyle, physical, medical and emotional aspects of this condition. They will address the questions you may have now and have not managed to ask anybody and they will address the questions you may have in the future, as you travel the many milestones of your individual diabetes life-cycle.

In this chapter I will take you through the following:

- What diabetes really is
- The various types of diabetes
- The 4 stages of progression in type 2 diabetes

These 3 sections will become the genesis of what we build on in this book henceforth.

Why is this chapter so important - When you look for information related to diabetes, you read what you find. Or somebody you know gives you an overview which may or may not make sense to you because it does not correspond to the stage of type 2 diabetes that you are in. This is because nobody tells you the story right from the beginning. <u>The first two chapters in this book are an attempt to explain the basics of diabetes in a sequential and streamlined fashion so that once and for all the entire picture is clear to you.</u> Also when you receive or seek more information in the future you know how to assimilate it and where to place it logically in your memory bank. The information here is also not exhaustive. It can't be because diabetes is being researched upon every single day. But it sure is a step in the right direction. Let's begin.

Let us start with understanding what hormones are - Hormones are chemical substances that act like messengers in the body. After being made in one part of the body, they travel to other parts of the body where they help control how cells and organs work for our bodies. This is where I can introduce insulin to you. <u>Insulin</u> is a hormone that is made in the beta cells of the pancreas. Insulin gets released in response to rising glucose in your bloodstream. After you eat a meal, the carbohydrates that you have eaten are broken down into glucose by the body and passed into your bloodstream. The pancreas detects this rise in blood glucose and secretes insulin.

So what role does insulin play - After you have a meal or a snack, the <u>pancreas</u> releases insulin. The insulin then signals muscle, fat and liver cells in your body to absorb the glucose (sugar) from the bloodstream to be used for energy. One can also understand insulin as a 'storage' hormone as it helps the body store excess glucose in the liver to be used at a later time. Insulin also signals the liver to stop releasing glucose into the bloodstream. Insulin helps shuttle amino acids (from protein digestion) and fatty acids (from fat digestion) into cells.

Understanding pancreas - The pancreas is an organ located in the abdomen. It plays an essential role in converting the food you eat into energy or fuel for the body's cells. The pancreas has two functions. One of them is called the endocrine function that regulates blood sugar. The endocrine component of the pancreas consists of islet cells that create and release important hormones directly into the bloodstream. Two of the main pancreatic hormones are insulin and glucagon. The beta cells in the pancreas secrete insulin and insulin acts to lower blood sugar. The alpha cells in the pancreas secrete glucagon and glucagon acts to raise blood sugar. Together they balance the body's blood sugars at healthy levels. When this does not happen, it leads to a condition called <u>diabetes.</u> Maintaining in-range blood sugar levels is critical in the functioning of key organs like the brain, liver and kidneys.

Now let's understand what diabetes really is - Diabetes mellitus is a group of metabolic or autoimmune disorders that affect how your body creates and / or uses blood sugar. As we just saw, glucose is important for your health as it is an important source of energy for the cells that make up your muscles and tissues. It is also your brain's main source of energy. No matter what <u>type of diabetes</u> you have, it can lead to excess sugar in your blood. Sustained periods of high blood sugar levels (hyperglycemia) can lead to serious health problems affecting one's eyes, heart, kidneys etc.

Let's now get to the various types of diabetes – There are many types of diabetes, but the 3 most common ones are:

Type 1 Diabetes is also called insulin-dependent diabetes. It used to be called juvenile-onset diabetes, as it used to often begin in childhood. Type 1 diabetes is an auto-immune condition. It happens when your body attacks your pancreas with antibodies. The organ is damaged and does not make insulin. Your genes might cause type 1 diabetes. It could also happen because of problems with cells in your pancreas that make insulin.

Type 2 Diabetes used to be called non-insulin-dependent or adult-onset diabetes. But over the last couple of decades it has become more common in children and teens. About 90% of people with diabetes have type 2 diabetes. When you have type 2 diabetes, your pancreas usually creates some insulin. But either it is not enough or your body does not use it like it should. Insulin resistance, when your cells don't respond to insulin, usually happens in fat, liver and muscle cells.

Pregnancy usually causes some form of insulin resistance. If this becomes diabetes, it is termed as **gestational diabetes.** Doctors often spot it in the middle or late pregnancy. Because the mother's blood sugars travel through the placenta to the baby, it is important to control gestational diabetes to protect the baby's growth and development. Gestational diabetes may go away after child birth. But in some women it can become type 2 diabetes weeks or even years later.

As you would have noted on the cover, this book is dedicated to type 2 diabetes. So let us now understand the **stages of progression** in type 2 diabetes.

Take a case in point. Rakesh was 40 when his doctor announced to him that he has type 2 diabetes. The diagnosis came up due to an annual corporate check-up at his organization. As in a lot of cases, Rakesh was surprised with the diagnosis. Today Rakesh is 52 years old and has gone through a few stages of type 2 diabetes. He started with metformin, the drug that is typically used as the first line of treatment. After 3 years, two more drugs were added to his list of anti-diabetics. These medicines did their job for 5 years after which Rakesh's doctor felt the need to put him on insulin. Like most type 2 diabetics Rakesh did not take this well. But his doctor went on to explain to him that this change was not Rakesh's fault. It was something that his body was doing and there was no other way of managing his diabetes.

Now this is probably something that we hear of day in and day out. Let's now understand why this was not Rakesh's fault and what really happened in his body. Diabetes is a progressive condition and often the first class of medicine is not sufficient for a very long period of time. One needs to move on to other classes of medicines and/or injectable.

The depletion and death of beta cells and insulin resistance - As we saw earlier, insulin is produced by beta cells in the pancreas. When the pancreas cannot produce enough insulin to regulate the blood sugar levels, it results in diabetes. The fundamental defect in type 2 diabetes is the inability of beta cells to make enough insulin for the body's needs. There are two factors at play. First the body becomes less sensitive to what insulin is trying to do and this is called insulin resistance. Second is to get the body's attention, the signal has to get stronger - which means the beta cells in the pancreas have to pump out more insulin and work harder. What changes is the beta cell response. At first, it improves to keep things normal in the face of insulin resistance. Unlike in people with type 1 diabetes, type 2 diabetics still have functioning beta cells in the early stage of diabetes. But usually they have no idea that their pancreas is struggling to keep up until a blood report flags high blood sugar levels. Most people on diagnosis have had diabetes for longer than they realise.

Because of their insulin resistance, people in the early stages of their diabetes may have highly functional beta cells - but not functional enough. In a person who is now officially diabetic, beta cell function may be twice what a non-diabetic individual has, but still not sufficient for that person. As long as there are functional beta cells in the body diabetes can be treated by attacking the body's insulin resistance.

But as the Rakesh example showed us, as time goes by metformin itself may not be enough. With insulin resistance as a prevailing issue, it becomes tough for the pancreas to sustain a level of hyper activity to secrete above-normal levels of insulin.
And then for reasons known and unknown, the function of beta cells worsens over time. They falter and fail as they stretch to pump out more and more insulin. This beta cell failure is responsible for what can feel like a 'life on a treadmill' for people with type 2 diabetes. The overload leads to progressive dysfunction.

Another way to represent this is the suggested staging model for type 2 diabetes:

Stage 1 Regulation of blood glucose is impaired and blood glucose is higher than normal. Diabetes complications may be present. <u>Haemoglobin A1c (HbA1c) 5.7-6.5%</u>

Stage 2 Ability to produce and use insulin is further impaired than Stage 1. Complications are often present, particularly in the circulatory and nervous systems. Metabolic syndrome is common. <u>HbA1c 6.5-9.0%</u>

Stage 3 Severe diabetic complications including neuropathy, vision loss, foot ulcers, amputation, blindness, kidney disease and heart disease. Hospitalisations may be frequent. <u>HbA1c above 9.0%</u>

Stage 4 Dangerously high glucose levels putting patients in danger of organ failure, highest chance of mortality. <u>HbA1c of 12% and/or diabetic emergencies</u>

**Now you know
why it was never your fault.**

I wanted to share this perspective to ensure that you banish the guilt and the stigma, if any, just because you developed type 2 diabetes. And if you are a caretaker to help you refrain from using negative words with your parent, spouse, sibling or child who is a diabetic. I will address the emotional aspects of diabetes later in the book in more detail.

Let us now address the reasons that are partially or completely in your control and paying heed may help you in delaying or in some cases helping you keep completely away from developing type 2 diabetes. Some of these reasons need getting rid of and some others extra care and sound medical advice:

You need to take extra care and get professional advice if you have:
- high blood pressure / high blood triglyceride levels and/ or low good cholesterol levels
- had gestational diabetes
- had / have pre-diabetes
- heart disease
- polycystic ovary syndrome (PCOS)

The habits that you need to get rid of or manage are:
- Smoking
- Unhealthy sleep patterns
- Alcohol
- Stress
- Unhealthy diet rich in refined sugars, carbohydrates and high fat content
- Being overweight
- Lack of exercise

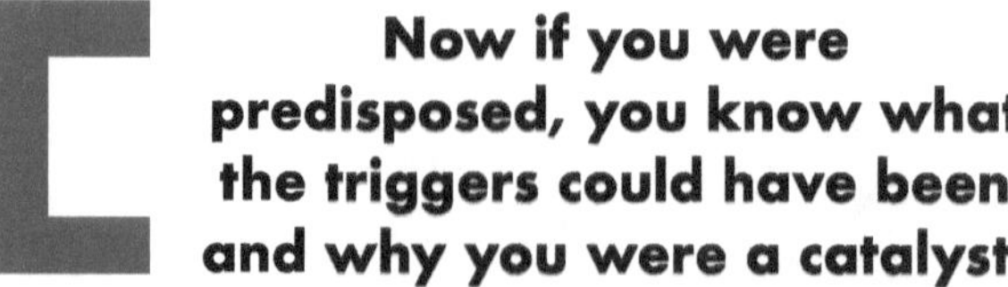

8 REASONS FOR HIGH BLOOD SUGAR LEVELS...

...understand the ominous octet

Now that you have warmed up to what diabetes really is, filled-in certain knowledge gaps, become aware of its various types and been cautioned about the multitude of complications it can lead to, it is important for you to also understand that <u>hyperglycemia or high blood sugar level is not a cause.</u> It is a symptom, a measure that tells us if somebody is diabetic or not. Like fever is a symptom for a certain infection. The main reasons for high blood sugar levels as we have learnt till date are lack of or insufficient insulin (because of damage to or depletion of beta cells - the source of insulin production in our bodies) and insulin resistance (the inability of the body to use this insulin). However, it is not necessarily that simple. <u>Type 2 diabetes actually contains 8 different defects in sugar metabolism that lead to high blood sugars. This has been referred to as the 'Ominous Octet'.</u> The 8 defects are shown in the figure in the following page.

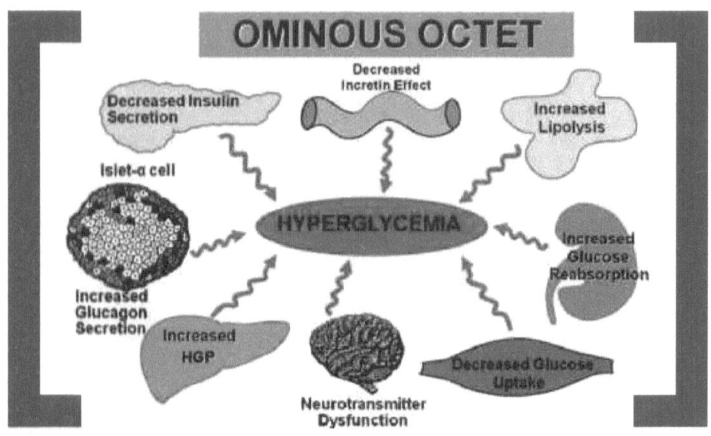

I am going to dedicate this chapter to explain this to you. These are facts that you may have never come across until now and unless you have an academic interest in this subject you may never get to this even in the future. Unfortunately these discussions rarely come up during a patient-doctor interaction. These interactions are largely limited to looking at reports and a change of dosage or medicines, unless there is a complication to deal with. **<u>But do you know why your doctor puts you on or pulls you off a certain class of diabetes medication? The reason is that there is a class of medication that correlates or corresponds to one or more of these 8 reasons for high blood sugar levels and attempts to compensate for them.</u>** This connection will get stronger as you reach chapter 6 that talks about the various classes of diabetes medications in detail. **<u>The reason for your diabetes and the medication/s thereof.</u>** For this very reason treat this as one of the most crucial chapters in this book.

Let us now go through the ominous octet one by one.

<u>1. Decreased insulin secretion</u> - Although insulin resistance typically causes increased amounts of insulin initially, these amounts are not enough to overcome the amount of glucose in the blood. The inability to correct blood sugars to normal levels is called impaired glucose tolerance (IGT). It has been found that once IGT is present, about 80% of pancreatic beta cell function has been lost. Further, over time, the remaining **pancreas** beta cells get "tired" and stop producing insulin altogether. This is why some type 2 diabetes patients become "insulin-dependent".

2. Decreased incretin effect - Another set of important hormones for glucose regulation are referred to as incretins. These are hormones that come from the **intestine**. The gut is made up of organs like your stomach and intestines. When you eat, incretins are released to help the body use glucose from the meal as well as suppressing your body from making more glucose. With type 2 diabetes, there is a decreased incretin effect in the body resulting in less insulin and increased blood sugar levels.

3. Increased lipolysis - This simply refers to increased fat breakdown. What is the problem with that, right? Well it's not the same as breaking down fat with exercise. **Fat cells** release more free fatty acids, and the excess lipid accumulates in liver (fatty liver), muscle and pancreas. This worsens overall insulin resistance and decreases insulin secretion. Just like muscle cells and liver cells, fat cells can be insulin resistant if you are overweight and / or have type 2 diabetes. This can cause high blood sugar levels.

4. Increased glucose reabsorption - The **kidney** has a remarkable ability to hold on to the glucose it filters, which is critical to providing for the energy demands of the body's tissues. In type 2 diabetes, the kidneys reabsorb too much sugar back into the blood, making it hard to keep blood sugar levels under control.

5. Decreased glucose uptake - **Muscle** cells have decreased ability to take up glucose and remove it from the bloodstream resulting in increased levels of glucose in your blood. Your muscles get their energy from sugar. But with type 2 diabetes, insulin has trouble moving sugar into muscle cells. This is called insulin resistance. When the body does not have enough insulin in the blood, it means glucose cannot get into muscles to fuel them. Over time, the lack of glucose can lead to muscle cells dying, resulting in the loss of muscle mass.

6. Neurotransmitter dysfunction - The <u>brain</u> plays an important role in glucose metabolism. Neurotransmitters are natural chemicals that stimulate the brain and nervous system. These signals are disrupted, and one of the major consequences is an increase in appetite. <u>This is likely why obesity and type 2 diabetes are highly correlated.</u> A part of the brain called the hypothalamus helps regulate how much you eat, affects your body's sensitivity to insulin, and affects how your body metabolises glucose and fats. In people with type 2 diabetes, changes in brain signaling can occur resulting in less of a response from signals, such as insulin, from the rest of the body.

7. Increased hepatic glucose production (HGP) - In times of need, the <u>liver</u> produces blood sugar through certain processes. This system goes unchecked in diabetes, where the liver continues to produce significant amounts of sugar, even when blood sugars are already high. If you have type 2 diabetes, your pancreas can release too much glucagon. This, in turn, causes the liver to release more sugar, leading to higher blood sugar levels.

8. Increased glucagon secretion - As we saw in chapter 1, the pancreas is where insulin is made. Insulin helps control blood sugar by moving sugar from the bloodstream into the body's cells for energy. The pancreas also makes the hormone glucagon. Glucagon tells the liver to release sugar into the blood to help balance blood sugar. With diabetes, the pancreas secretes less insulin and more glucagon which can contribute to higher blood sugar levels.

Another way of looking at the ominous octet is by understanding the body parts that contribute to the progression of type 2 diabetes. The image below represents it beautifully. In each of the reasons above I have made the connection to the respective body part by highlighting the corresponding word...pancreas, intestine, fat cells, kidneys, muscle cells, the brain and liver.

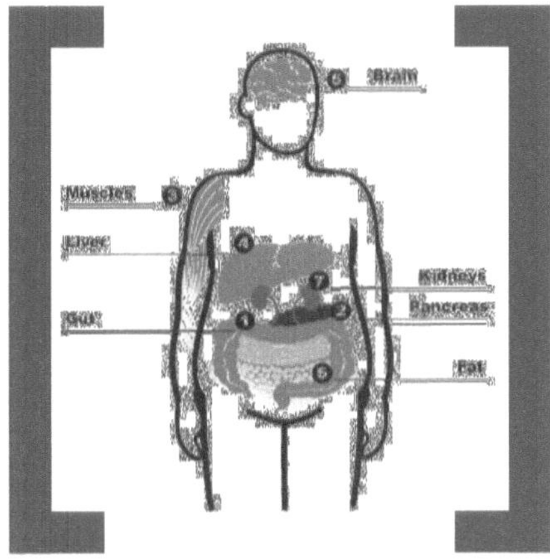

As I have explained earlier, the identification of these 8 defects has significant implications for treating type 2 diabetes. The attempt that our doctors make is to attack diabetes from multiple angles. This also tells us that type 2 diabetes should be treated in a comprehensive fashion and not from only a single point-of-view. Metformin which is one of the most popular medicines is a great medication to be on, as long as it is tolerated, as it takes care of 2 of these reasons.

As the science behind diabetes unfolded, there were many more factors that got added to the ominous octet. This led to further addition of factors that resulted in glucose intolerance, thus extending the ominous octet to the 'dirty dozen', the 'treacherous thirteen' and the 'formative fifteen'.

I am conscious of the fact that chapters 1 and 2 have turned out a little more technical than I would have liked them to be. The reason is simple. The more you understand about the basics of diabetes, the more you know that there are a zillion things that are not in our control. This further emphasises the importance of the 3 basic variables that are in our control. Our food, how we exercise and the medications we take. And most importantly how we adhere to them in our constant attempt to compensate for what nature took away from us.

CHAPTER EXERCISE

In the diabetes context, match the following from what we have learnt so far:

Body Part	Function
1. Brain	A. Tells the liver to release sugar to balance blood sugar levels
2. Beta cells	B. Produce insulin
3. Glucagon	C. Helps in moving glucose from bloodstream into cells
4. Insulin	D. Produce glucagon
5. Alpha cells	E. End up reabsorbing too much glucose leading to hyperglycemia
6. Kidneys	F. Sends signals that affect your body's sensitivity to insulin

Answers: *1-F, 2-B, 3-A, 4-C, 5-D, 6-E*

STIMULATE YOURMIRR ORNEURO NS

STIMULATE YOUR MIRROR NEURONS...

03 **...the key to understanding overeating and obesity**

When you see your friend hurting herself you flinch in sympathy. When you see a person's facial expression while tasting something you tend to react in a similar manner. A happy expression makes you eager to taste that food and a wrinkled face makes you think twice about tasting it. This ability to instinctively and immediately understand what other people are experiencing has long baffled neuroscientists, but recent research now suggests a fascinating explanation: **brain cells called mirror neurons.** Mirror neurons are a special class of brain cells that fire not only when an individual performs an action, but also when the individual observes someone else making the same movement. This has radically altered the way we think about our brains and ourselves, particularly our social selves.

Before the discovery of mirror neurons, scientists generally believed that our brains use logical thought processes to interpret and predict other people's actions. Now, however, many have come to believe that **we understand others not by thinking, but by feeling.** This is because mirror neurons appear to let us "simulate" not just other people's actions, but the intentions and emotions behind those actions. When you see someone smile, your mirror neurons for smiling fire up too, creating a sensation in your own mind of the feeling associated with smiling. You don't have to think about what the other person intends by smiling. You experience the meaning immediately and effortlessly.

Mirror neurons are how we mimic others. Children typically mimic adults as a way of acquiring adult behaviours and actions. This mimicking behaviour continues throughout life, and people tend to automatically mimic the expressions, body language, and behaviours of others, often without the knowledge that they are doing that.

People mimic the eating behaviours of others too, including choices of food and portions.

This also leads people to prefer the foods favoured by others whose eating behaviour they have mimicked. One study has suggested that obesity is contagious within social networks and mirror neurons could be the mechanism through which this is possible. Mimicking represents an independent neurophysiological pathway to stimulate overeating.

Food is the genesis of our lives. I don't mean it as a means of survival or as a necessity for growth and development. Food is a relationship. When we sit down and share a meal with someone, we form a special bond with them. Not because of what we spoke about, but because of what we shared from a plate.

Food is an emotion. It makes us happy. In some ways our moods dictate what we eat and in other ways what we eat dictates our moods. Food comforts us, cajoles us and loves us like nothing else. Food for us is our mothers. It is the fulcrum on which our childhoods and all our memories are anchored on. Some foods remind us of our fathers because they were the ones who introduced us to them. Others bring up associations - of childhood buddies, school friends and cousins.

Food is an occasion. It has and will always remain celebratory. Maybe it was a meal with someone special. Or was it a festival and a special cuisine thereof. Food for us is an experience. Of the places we visited. Their unique blends and preparations.

Food is also transient. It either defines us or gets defined by our life stage. My food has changed over years. It has transitioned from being home-cooked, benign and nutritious, to exploratory and daring and then settling back to caution when I entered the fourth decade of my life.

During the latter half of my 3rd decade, I was told that this precious food was one of the main reasons for my ill health and that I had to change my habits to be able to lead a healthier life. It destroyed me mentally, emotionally and in every which way possible. I was a wreck. It was like someone had pulled away my mental crutch and was asking me to walk on one leg. The 36th year of my life was a turning point. I was proclaimed a type 2 diabetic with postprandial readings of more than 300 and an HbA1c of 10.

At that time I did not understand the science of food. I did not understand words like the global obesity epidemic, excessive food consumption, automatic reflexive response, increased caloric intake and the inter-relation between obesity and type 2 diabetes. I did not know that a global obesity epidemic is increasing with increase in the availability and salience of food in the environment.

I didn't know that obesity is increasing across all socioeconomic groups and educational levels and occurs even among individuals with the highest levels of education and expertise in nutrition and related fields. I didn't know that the current food environment stimulates automatic reflexive responses that enhance the desire to eat and increase caloric intake, making it exceedingly difficult for individuals like me to resist, especially because I may not be aware of these influences. And I definitely didn't know about mirror neurons.

I am sure you are much more aware than I was. But I started reading and I never stopped. It changed my understanding of food. I understood about food classifications that matter. I understood the correlation between healthy blood sugar levels and foods. I understood about refined and processed foods and I understood about dietary fiber. What I am sharing below is an abstract from the American Diabetes Association along with my own notes that correlate to food environments that I am aware of. You may entirely or partially relate. But relate you will and it will help you rationalise what you already know better.

There are 10 neurophysiological pathways that can lead us to make food choices subconsciously or, in some cases, automatically. These pathways include reflexive and uncontrollable neurohormonal responses to food images, cues, and smells; mirror neurons that cause us to imitate the eating behaviour of others without awareness; and our limited cognitive capacity to make informed decisions about food. Further, we have a limited ability to shape the food environment around us and no ability to control automatic responses to food-related cues that are unconsciously perceived.

In simple terms, below are the 10 human characteristics that are used by food marketers world-over to exploit our food related behaviours.

CHARACTERISTIC 1	MECHANISM	HOW IT IS EXPLOITED
Our physiological response to food and to images of food	Dopamine is secreted when food is perceived and dopamine creates motivations for food	Food is all around us. And if not food itself, its images. On TV, in malls, on the street, everywhere. Food is omnipresent.

This is what you should know: Dopamine is a feel-good hormone and an important part of our brain's reward system. Eating junk food causes release of dopamine in the brain. This reward encourages susceptible individuals like us to eat more unhealthy foods. To add to this, frequent consumption of junk food may lead to dopamine tolerance. This means that you will have to eat a higher amount of junk food to avoid going into withdrawal. It is very similar to smoking or alcohol consumption patterns.

Cravings will appear out of thin air. You may be watching a movie, reading, listening to music or on a call. The craving for wafers, a burger, a soft drink or an ice-cream will appear out of nowhere. Have you experienced this? Such cravings can also be attributed to certain triggers called cues. These cues can be as simple as walking past an ice cream shop or your favourite pizza outlet. An ad, a smell, content marketing or a brand tune can trigger it. A true craving is about satisfying the brain's need for dopamine. It has nothing to with the body's need for energy or nourishment. Regularly giving in to cravings for junk food may be a sign that you are experiencing food addiction or emotional eating.

<table>
<tr><td>CHARACTERISTIC 2</td><td>MECHANISM</td><td>HOW IT IS EXPLOITED</td></tr>
<tr><td>Our inborn preferences for sugar and fat</td><td>Under stress, we choose items that provide immediate calories to respond to increased energy demands</td><td>Excessive availability and production of cheap energy-dense, high-fat and high-sugar content foods</td></tr>
</table>

This is what you should know: Eating seems to be a predominant solution to all our problems. We eat when we are happy and we eat when we are stressed. But it is important to understand that stress and eating can be a deadly combination, especially for people like us. Our bodies respond to stress by increasing levels of cortisol, which gets the body ready to "fight or flee". Cortisol, a stress hormone released by the adrenal glands, increases in response to a threat. When you no longer perceive a threat, cortisol levels return to normal. But if stress is a permanent feature of your life (personal, professional or both) then you can experience an overexposure to cortisol. Now cortisol is also a significant appetite stimulant. That is how stress and appetite go hand in hand and that is why so many people respond to stress by going for comfort foods and end up having a whole pack of chips or an ice-cream tub. The risks of stress and weight gain are hypertension and diabetes, just to name a few.

CHARACTERISTIC 3	MECHANISM	HOW IT IS EXPLOITED
Our hardwired survival strategies	We automatically respond to abundance and variety by consuming more	The marketing efforts of organizations, malls and supermarkets to increase shelf space and the abundant display of high-calorie foodstuffs; increased introduction of product varieties with empty calories and zero nutritional values

This is what you should know: Human beings evolved as hunters-gatherers. Today's food industry has been extremely savvy in exploiting both scarcity and abundance to make us buy more and eventually consume more, much more than what we need. Scarcity is still being exploited by certain environments by asking customers to pick up 'not more than X nos. of something. Research shows that limiting supply of items (say a 'maximum of 5 per customer'), even if there is no change to pricing, drives scarcity considerations and actually serves to increase demand for products. Our survival instincts kick-in. Our brains are hard-wired to perceive and seek scarce resources. After the initial days of supply chains genuinely getting affected due to covid-19, many marketers exploited this emotion to the hilt in the year 2020.

On the other hand abundance is another factor that is used to make consumers buy more. Do you now understand why shelves in supermarkets are arranged the way they are. Why are there so many food products kept in the check-out zones? And why did buffets and brunches become so popular? But when these purchases and indulgence leads to undue high calorie consumption of nutrient-deficit foods, the story turns towards obesity, metabolic diseases and ill health. The United Kingdom is bringing in a law to stop marketers and restaurants from luring vulnerable customers into buying more unhealthy snacks and consuming more sugary drinks. This law is due to come into effect from April 2021. Food environments around us will see positive changes. Till then and beyond, we have to take care of ourselves.

CHARACTERISTIC 4	MECHANISM	HOW IT IS EXPLOITED
Our inability to judge calorie content	Visual system cannot judge volume or content; signals of satiety are imprecise, based more on volume than energy density	Excessively large portion sizes are available in packaged goods as well as in restaurants

This is what you should know: It is human nature to eat when presented with food, and to eat more when presented with more food. The trouble is that we are pushed more food, more often, every day. In fact, it seems that the only people who are immune to big portions are tiny children. Up until the age of three or four, children have an enviable ability to stop eating when they are full. After that age, this self-regulation of hunger is lost, and sometimes never relearned. Even in a country like India where traditional cooking still exists, the modern kitchen has lost its basic instincts about cooking. Conventional wisdom and the number on your glucometer can provide you the much needed guideline. Without these self-developed calibrations, you will remain at the mercy of the food industry.

In a state of overabundance, food companies have two possible strategies. One is to sell us smaller portions at higher prices, which you and I are conditioned to perceive as a loss. The other, more universal approach is to attempt to sell us more food which we know is very easily done. In India, one way out is to shop from the traditional 'kirana' stores that do not have enough square-feet of display space. These mom and pop stores also take orders on the phone and deliver your grocery right to your homes. This will help reduce unnecessary exposure to tempting supermarket triggers and reduce unhealthy indulgence. If you don't bring it home, you will not have it.

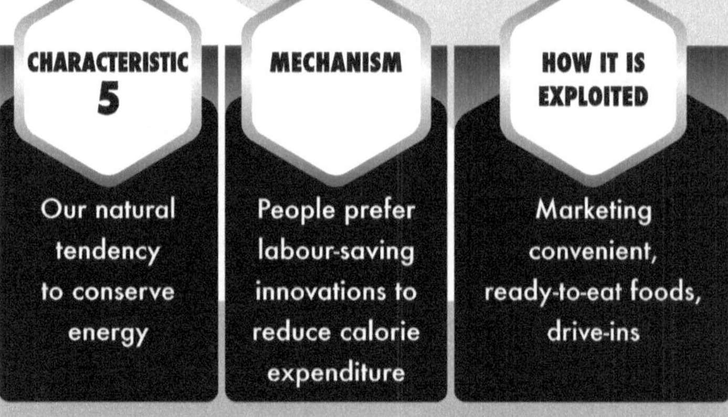

This is what you should know: Besides being hardwired about our responses to food, we are also hardwired with respect to conserving energy through shortcuts. This means that we are automatically more attracted to food that is convenient compared with food that requires work to prepare. Marketers have tried to capitalise on this tendency by developing products that make eating quick and easy, including packaging that allows people to eat on the run, eat in their cars, and eat with only one hand. Easy home-delivery mechanisms have only added to this natural in-built laziness. The concept of whole foods, foods with high fibre content, home-cooked food and foods that are closest to their original selves (minimal processing and refining) are making a comeback, albeit slowly, to help fight lifestyle and other metabolic diseases.

CHARACTERISTIC 6	MECHANISM	HOW IT IS EXPLOITED
Mirror neurons	People unconsciously mimic others' eating behaviours	Modeling eating behaviors

This is what you should know: We have seen the relevant explanation to this in the 3rd paragraph of this chapter. What I would like to add here is that since children mimic eating behaviours of adults, especially their parents, the onus is on the parents to help their children model the right kind of behaviour. This would not only include adoption of 'mindful' eating behaviour by parents, but also extend to helping the child model buying behaviours with respect to grocery and food items. We will talk about 'mindful eating' in the next chapter.

This is what you should know: Human beings are conditioned to respond to brand perceptions, symbols, status and imagery. Marketers exploit this tendency through the use of branding—a name, term, design, symbol, or other features to distinguish one product or service from competitive offerings. Over time, we the customers learn to buy the brand rather than the product. The brand becomes the shortcut that motivates actions like purchase or consumption.

Prices also guide the choices that we make on food consumption. Prices play a role in the kinds of foods that are consumed, with people eating more of less expensive energy-dense items than more expensive, nutrient-rich items like fruits and vegetables. Nevertheless, in many places, the status associated with a product may be more important than price in determining consumption. In many cultures, people will purchase items perceived to be associated with high status items, such as sugar-sweetened beverages, and forego less expensive but more nutritious items like natural coconut water.

As a consequence of the current food environment, in countries undergoing the "nutrition transition," many children with nutrient-poor diets become stunted at the same time as the adults in the household are becoming obese. This may typically happen in economies that are starting to have higher disposable incomes. Food choices are not occurring at the level of rational decision-making, but are governed by the impulsive, emotional, and non-rational parts of our brain simply because of the way foods are marketed.

CHARACTERISTIC 8	MECHANISM	HOW IT IS EXPLOITED
Priming	Automatically respond to items made salient through indirect methods	Use of music, lighting, images, symbols, to enhance purchase of foods

This is what you should know: Priming is another technique that marketers use to influence food purchases and to increase consumption. It is used to evoke specific memories or associations that make a person more disposed to act in a particular way. Just as violent television programs can prime children to be more aggressive and violent, images, sounds, smells, and even lighting prime people to be hungry or desire food. One study pointed out that customers were more likely to buy French wines when a liquor store played French music and more likely to purchase German wines when German music was played. We usually do not recognise the prime and, even when we are aware of it, we usually do not realise that our behaviour is influenced by the prime. In fact, most of us deny that we are influenced by images or advertising, even though we think others are.

CHARACTERISTIC 9	MECHANISM	HOW IT IS EXPLOITED
Automatic stereotype activation	Automatic responses to items that are associated with the self and with social groups and expectations	Use of racial/ethnic groups and celebrities to model eating behaviours

This is what you should know: Eating behaviours may also be influenced by automatic responses to stereotypes. We know that people respond to others based on stereotypes and that the responses are not conscious. We also know that we have greater empathy and trust in people who look like us and are wary when confronted with others who appear different. Advertisers exploit the fact that we respond more favourably to images of people like ourselves and now customise their marketing / advertising to reflect the appearance of the target groups. It is called customer segmentation in marketing terms and used throughout the world by fast-food brands very successfully.

<table>
<tr><th>CHARACTERISTIC
10</th><th>MECHANISM</th><th>HOW IT IS
EXPLOITED</th></tr>
<tr><td>Limited cognitive capacity</td><td>People can be distracted or overwhelmed with too much information and influenced to eat impulsively or make unwise dietary choices</td><td>Lack of labeling or warnings, or use of confusing and inaccurate labels; e.g. "no cholesterol" labels on foods that are high in sugar and salt</td></tr>
</table>

This is what you should know: We can only process a limited amount of information at one time; when we are overloaded, we tend to make decisions impulsively. We typically choose the default option that requires no processing demands. When it comes to food too this logic applies and the default options unfortunately are the most omnipresent items high in sugar and fat.

Now you know how you should shop for food. Now you also know that you should consciously attempt to resist the omnipresent triggers around you that make you and your family buy more and consume more.

Let us in the next chapter understand the food classifications that really matter. The contents of the next chapter may as well appear in secondary school syllabi and help condition our future generations to a healthier way of thinking about food.

CHAPTER EXERCISE

Match the following from what we have learnt so far:

A	B
1. Dopamine	A. Is a stress hormone
2. Cortisol	B. Showing same race or ethnicity in a burger advertisement
3. Mirror Neurons	C. Is a feel good hormone
4. Automatic Stereotype Activation	D. Use of sound, lights etc to make us buy
5. Priming	E. Exploited to easy and economical home-deliveries
6. Natural tendency to conserve energy	F. Is why we mimic other behaviours

Answers: 1-C, 2-A, 3-F, 4-B, 5-D, 6-E

FOCUS ON FOOD...

04 ...and change your paradigm

In the previous chapter we understood the food responses we are inherently born with and the added stimuli that the food environment around us provides, thus endangering our lives as far as increased calorie consumption and acceleration towards severe diabetes complications go. In medical terms, managing food habits to attain better glycaemic control is called 'medical nutritional therapy'. You will be surprised and happy to know that medical nutritional therapy (food) interventions have helped in decreasing HbA1cs in the range of 0.5% to 2.6%. This is in fact more than or equivalent to the positive effect of many glucose-lowering medications as you will see in chapter 6. That is why a changed perspective on food is so important and I attempt to give you that in this chapter.

Earlier it was widely believed that blood glucose response to different diets is determined mainly by the amount of carbohydrate they contain. There was no differentiation made between various carbohydrates. The concept of glycaemic index (GI) classifies the blood glucose-raising potential of carbohydrate foods. This has shown that foods with <u>similar</u> carbohydrate contents <u>did not</u> usually have the same impact on blood glucose levels.

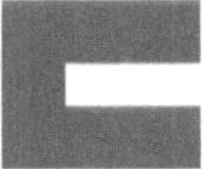 **This also means that all carbohydrates are not made equal.** 

Given this critical information, the concept of glycaemic index has revolutionised the world of diet-planning for diabetics and further transformed itself into a key player for the prevention and management of diabetes. I personally follow this in my diet plan. I have moved away from wheat, white rice and refined flour as my main carbohydrate sources and adopted brown rice. The glycaemic index of white rice is around 70 and that of brown rice around 50. Other food items remaining the same (a low GI vegetable, some form of dal and curd), my postprandial readings are in the range of 125 to 140 when I have brown rice, versus readings of close to 160 when it is white rice. I have now mastered the art of portion control too. My treats are chapatis (rotis) and I have them only twice a week. I deliberately choose low glycaemic index fruits over the high glycaemic index ones on a regular basis. Having said that, let us appreciate the fact that this does not mean that I have blacklisted certain food items or kept them aside as 'foods to avoid' forever due to their high glycaemic index. I have them, but once in a way. This is where common sense chips in.

Let us now understand what glycaemic index is
Carbohydrate is an essential part of our diets, but not all carbohydrate foods are equal. The glycaemic index (GI) is a relative ranking of carbohydrates in foods according to how they affect blood glucose levels. Carbohydrates with a low GI value (55 or less) are more slowly digested, absorbed and metabolised and cause a lower and slower rise in blood glucose. This also means that you do not feel hungry again for that much longer. The chart on the following page explains it well.

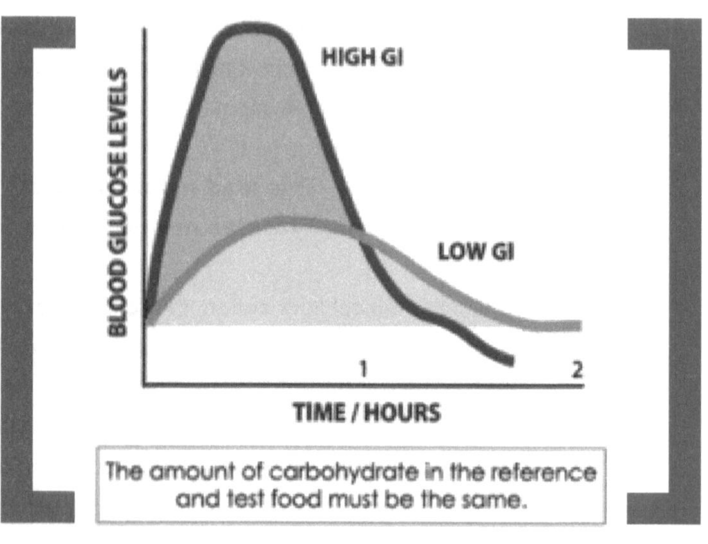

There are three classifications for individual food portion GI:

	Low GI	Mid GI	High GI
	55 or less	56 - 69	70 +

So what is glycaemic load?

Your blood glucose levels rise and fall when you eat a meal containing carbohydrates. How high it rises and how long it stays high depends on the quality of the carbohydrates (the GI) as well as the quantity. Glycaemic load (or GL) combines both the quantity and quality of carbohydrates. It is also the best way to compare blood glucose values of different types and amounts of foods. The formula for calculating the glycaemic load of a particular food or meal is:

Glycaemic Load
= GI x
Carbohydrate (g)
content per portion
÷ 100.

<u>**Let's look at it with the following examples:**</u>

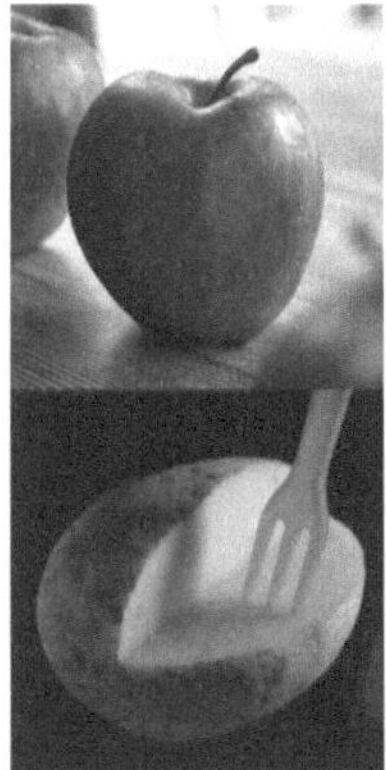

A single apple has a GI of 38 and contains 13 grams of carbohydrates.
Hence GL = 38 x 13/100 = 5

• •

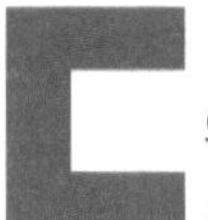

A potato has a GI of 85 and contains 14 grams of carbohydrates.
Hence GL=85 x 14 /100 = 12

<u>We can therefore safely say that</u>
<u>a potato will have more than twice the</u>
<u>glycaemic effect than that of an apple.</u>

Similar to the glycaemic index, the glycaemic load of a food can be classified as low, medium, or high:

Low GL	Mid GL	High GL
10 or less	11-19	20 +

Now let us understand which one to use in the practical sense

Although the GL concept has been useful in scientific research, it's the GI that's proven most helpful to people with diabetes and those who are overweight. That's because a diet with a low GL, unfortunately, can be a 'mixed bag'. It can be full of healthy low GI carbs in some cases, but also too high in protein in others or low in carbs and full of the wrong sorts of fats (i.e., saturated) such as those found in some 'discretionary foods'.

If you use the GI as it was originally intended – to choose the lower GI option within a food group or category – you usually end-up selecting the one with the lowest GL anyway because foods are grouped together for a reason because they contain similar nutrients, including amounts of carbohydrate. So, if you choose healthy low GI foods, at least one at each meal, chances are you're eating a diet that not only keeps blood glucose in a healthy range but also helps you achieve that with a balanced nutrition.

Now you can start using the internet (credible sites) to draw your list of foods and note down their respective GIs.

While we may not use GL in our diet planning as much as we may use GI, it may still help to understand how they work together, especially in deciding how we consume various food items. Let's take 4 examples:

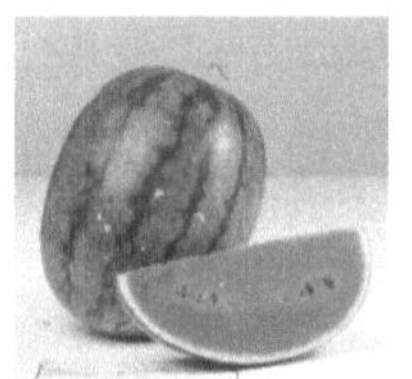

Watermelon has a high GI of 72, yet a low GL of 7.21.
The high GI is based on 5 cups of watermelon, not an actual serving size of 1 cup.
The low GL means one serving of watermelon doesn't contain much carbohydrate, because it is actually mostly water.
The low GL indicates that a serving of watermelon won't have much impact on your blood sugar.
Lesson - eat in moderate quantities

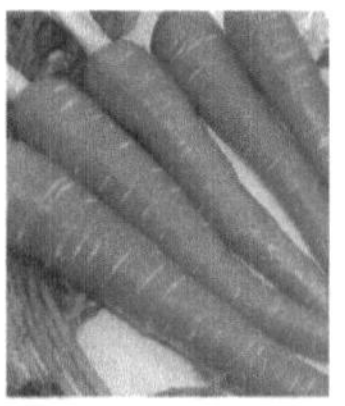

Carrots are another example of a low GL food that many people think will raise their blood sugar a lot – but it's not true.
The perception is due to their high GI of 71.
However, what most people don't know is that the GL for carrots is only 6.
Lesson - unless you're going to eat a kilo of carrots in one sitting, an average serving of carrots will have very little impact on blood glucose level.
The same holds true for beetroot too. GI – 65, GL – 5.

<u>**Now look at a carbohydrate example to understand portion sizes once again:**</u>

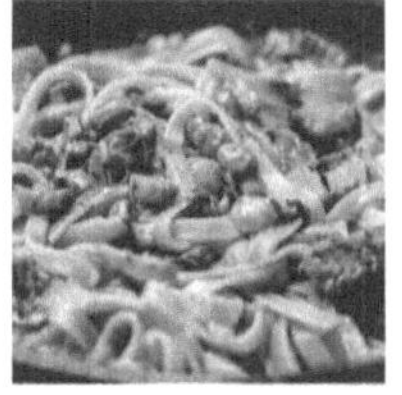

GI of a standard white wheat pasta, not over-cooked = 43

The carbohydrate content of a standard 180g serve = 44g

GL = 43 x 44/100 = 19g (mid GL)

However, if only half a portion of pasta was eaten, the GL would also halve given that GI is still 43

The carbohydrate content of a half portion 90g serve = 22g

GL = 43 x 22/100 = 9.5g

<u>Lesson - learn portion control</u>

· ·

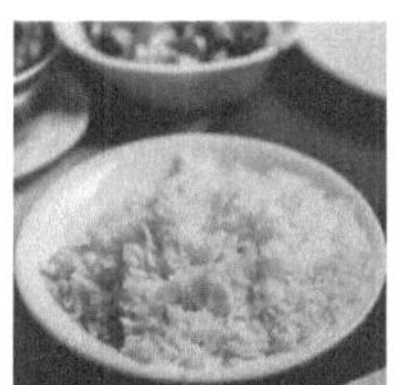

A study demonstrated that cooling of cooked white rice increased its resistant starch content making it relatively better for diabetics.

Cooked white rice cooled at 4°C for 24 hours then reheated had higher resistance starch content than cooked white rice cooled at room temperature for 10 hours.

In the clinical study, ingestion of cooked white rice cooled at 4°C for 24 hours then reheated produced a lower glycaemic response compared with ingestion of freshly cooked white rice at the same portion.

Cooked white rice cooled at 4°C (which is what our refrigerator temperatures normally are) for 24 hours then reheated was also accepted nearly as well as freshly cooked white rice.

Therefore, changing freshly cooked white rice to cooked white rice cooled at 4°C for 24 hours then reheated can be recommended for diabetic patients in everyday diet.

<u>**Lesson - foods high in resistant starch are better for diabetics**</u>

http://apjcn.nhri.org.tw/server/APJCN/24/4/620.pdf

· ·

There are many other lessons that you will learn as you go down this path. Most importantly, once you have the focus, the learning will happen automatically.

So where do we go wrong?

With respect to fruits and vegetables:

- We tend to have very large portions.

    I have seen some people have half a large melon or a few mangoes at one go. Imagine what happens to our bodies when we have a fruit salad as dessert after a meal. The amount of calorie intake is grossly harmful. Or when we have potatoes as our main vegetable with rotis or rice. Carbohydrate + carbohydrate is a harmful combination.

- We have fruits immediately after food which results in disproportionately high calorie intake for a meal.

    Fruits are a snack and they should be eaten in isolation. Not before or after a meal.

- We juice fruits and vegetables and thereby consume large amounts of it.

    Some people add sugar to it and make it toxic for type 2 diabetics.

- We consume soups made of high GI vegetables in large quantities as the first course of a meal.

    The concept of 3-course or 4-course meals invariably makes us consume too much for a single meal.

    Keep away from buffets.

    Also while juices and soups have vitamins and minerals, they are bereft of the fibre that whole fruits and vegetables have. Fibre is important for the regulation of blood sugar spikes.

- We tend to have overripe versions of fruits because they are sweeter.

    As a fruit ripens, its GI increases.

With respect to a carbohydrate:

- We eat very large portions

    As Indians we find it difficult to have a meal without a

carbohydrate. In our minds our meals are incomplete
without them. In fact carbohydrates anchor all our meals
and most of our snacks. This is the biggest mistake that we
make as a country.

- We overcook them resulting in an increase in their GI.
  For example overcooked pasta has a higher glycaemic index
  than pasta that is neither over nor under cooked. Mashed
  potatoes have a higher GI than baked potatoes. We have also
  understood the importance of resistant starch in this context.

You can bring down the overall glycaemic index of a meal by
combining a high glycaemic index food with foods that have lower
ones. Your age, how active you are, and how fast you digest food
will also affect how your body reacts to carbohydrates.

A well balanced meal with moderate portions is the way to go.
Your glucometer will ultimately decide the meal combinations and
the portion sizes that are ideal for you. (Reference - Chapter 9).

So what is glycaemic response

After eating a meal, the digestible or available carbohydrates are
absorbed into the bloodstream, producing an increase in blood
glucose concentration. In time the blood glucose concentration falls
back to or below fasting levels. The magnitude of the rise and fall
of blood glucose and the duration over which it occurs has been
termed the glycaemic response. More slowly digestible
carbohydrates or minimally processed starchy foods produce a
different response. Compared with rapidly digestible
carbohydrates they show a slower and more prolonged increase in
blood glucose, rising to a lower peak. Other factors include how
much food you eat, how much the food is processed and even how
the food is prepared, For example, pasta that is cooked so that it is
still firm when bitten has a slower glycaemic response than pasta
that is overcooked. The ripeness of a fruit can change its glycaemic
response. A less ripe banana will have a slower glycaemic
response than an over ripe banana.

Finally, you may have known these concepts earlier, but not looked at them in this context or you may not have known of them. Either way, do not worry about remembering everything you just read. Don't be overwhelmed. Just keep them at the back of your mind as a reference point. Slowly and steadily, as you adopt this way of eating, you will internalise it all. How to implement this to create your new food plan and to make your own good-food universe is in chapter 9. It may be a good idea to go directly to chapter 9 from here to understand how to put them to use together.

Mindful eating

A lot has been said about mindful eating. But the reason that I have brought it up here is because it is the antithesis to all the 10 ways we are manipulated in, to buy and eat more, as we saw in the earlier chapter. <u>It is the antidote to most of our inborn biases towards food and the negative external stimuli that make us gravitate towards food that much more.</u> The solution is within us. Mindful eating will help us fight these triggers by being aware, conscious and deliberate about our food-related behaviours.

So how do we eat in this manner? For each one of us mindful eating will begin the day we start eating food with a complete sense of awareness. Mindful eating will begin the day we stop treating food as a pass-time, a distraction, something to fill our boredoms with or to munch on while watching TV. Food actually is a weapon that is going to not only save our lives, but also help us reach our peaks physically and emotionally. It will begin the day we start treating our bodies and our food with the respect they deserve. Fundamentally, mindful eating involves:

- eating slowly and without distraction
- listening to physical hunger cues and eating only until you're full
- distinguishing between true hunger and non-hunger triggers for eating
- engaging your senses by noticing colours, smells, sounds, textures and flavours
- learning to cope with guilt and anxiety about food
- eating to maintain overall health and well-being

- noticing the effects food has on your feelings and other parameters
- appreciating your food

Start practicing mindful eating along with your newfound diet. It is a winning combination and will do wonders to the way the diet works for you, glycaemic control-wise.

On a lighter note, here is something I have experienced at South Indian weddings. It brings out our excesses as human beings and our total disregard for our bodies and our physical and emotional health. Enjoy the read...

Once I turned diabetic, I understood what white rice does to the human body. Its high glycaemic index increases blood sugar faster than it should, even if consumed in very limited quantities. Now in this context, the icing on the cake is a South Indian wedding, especially the ones in Tamil Nadu or Palakkad. These weddings are well known for their grand 5-course meals on a banana leaf. Unfortunately for a diabetic and every human being who is health conscious, every course is RICE.

The first course is dal & rice with ghee and the caterers almost tease you with the super-micro quantity they serve during this course. The next course is sambar & rice and this you thoroughly do enjoy. But even before you finish half of what has been served and relish it, a fresh attack is launched at you and a new wave of rice is served, now with rasam. By this time the enjoyment turns into a mild of form of fear. The amount of rice in your banana leaf is unnerving. Each serving is a small mountain of rice that one needs to climb. Anybody who has been to a South Indian wedding will vouch for this unsettling phenomenon.

At this stage the caterers decide that it's time to take you through a small detour and you are served with kheer, which again turns out to be sweetened rice and milk. This stage is tricky. Even though you are completely full and even a single morsel would seem impossible, you tend to consume a few glasses of it. That is the unavoidable magic of the South Indian Payasam. And finally when your body and your mind separate just because of the sheer amount of rice and sugar in your body, comes the final blow... more rice and buttermilk.

I have been to these weddings when I was a non-diabetic. And I enjoyed this bodily crime voluntarily. But in my last 14 years as a diabetic, I went to only one poonal (a thread ceremony). The food served here is similar to what is served during weddings. Despite knowing everything I needed to know about the negatives of rice and sugar, I got swept away and managed to get my sugar levels to around 300. In my personal experience certain foods can take your sugar levels high, but the fall back to normal levels is reasonably quick. But when you consume the most chronic combination of an inhuman amount of rice and sugar, nothing in this world can help you. It will take hours before your sugar levels get to normal. This is 100% inclusive of immense fatigue and high levels of guilt.

One can't avoid going to weddings and poonals. But the one piece of advice I want to leave you with is to stay absolutely away from the hot and sweaty food zones and enjoy an apple and some buttermilk in the air-conditioned hall. And if you have been disciplined and want to enjoy some of that food, have a glass of that payasam, say a premature goodbye to your cousins and hit the gym.

CHAPTER EXERCISE

Match the following from what we have learnt so far:

A	B
1. Low GI range	A. The rate at which sugar levels go up as a response to carbohydrate consumption
2. Low GL range	B. 55 or less
3. This takes into consideration carbohydrate content	C. Helps us to make rational choices about eating
4. Mindful eating	D. 10 or less
5. Before GI was introduced	E. Glycaemic Load
6. GI is	F. All carbohydrates were considered equal

Answers: 1-B, 2-D, 3-E, 4-C, 5-F, 6-A

A WALK
CAN BE
MAGICAL...

A WALK CAN BE MAGICAL...

05

...use it as a strategic weapon

This is going to be the shortest chapter in this book. After getting your perspective on food right, it is now time to tackle the second variable - burning calories. In fact the chapters in this book flow in the same sequence as I considered these variables and implemented them for myself. In the next chapter we will talk about medication, the third variable.

I would like you to appreciate that when I talk about walking, I am going to talk about it with only one objective in mind - to help you achieve the HbA1c goals you have set for yourself. Also, don't be discouraged. I am not going to give you the same old tricks and tips that every other article on walking gives you. I am not going to talk to you about the kind of footwear you should have and neither am I going to talk to you about the various apps or techniques regarding walking. I am going to talk to you about 2 very focused things: 1. The timing of your walk and 2. The quantum of your walk

A small personal experience on walking before I get to that.

During my sabbatical in 2014, the first major change that I made was to my food universe. I measured my blood glucose levels after every meal and noted it. At the end of 14 days I had eliminated what was taking me over 150 and noting down what worked for me. Finally I had a calendar that told me what suits my body, in what quantities should I have it and at what times of the day. Before I started this routine I weighed 80 kilos and had an a1c of over 8.5 for very many years.

But once I began, in a month or so, purely with the help of my new diet, I lost around 3 kilos. Some of you may understand this feeling of exuberance. Instead of 8, I had a 7 as the first number for my weight. This feeling motivated me to add some form of physical exercise to my effort. I started walking in the mornings. On my very first day, I walked for 20 minutes and I felt jubilant. The endorphins did their job well and I started feeling good after my walks. After the initial feeling of irrational happiness my mind turned logical and surveyed the track I had available for walking. There was this squarish perimeter that I wanted to measure. The next sets of activities were a drain on my pocket but worth my while. I got myself all the relevant gear, including shoes, socks, track pants and tons of t-shirts. Good, stylish and trendy gear always add a lot of motivation to any activity, at least initially. The perimeter measured around 1.5 kms and It took me 20 minutes on day one. Now I manage that in 12 minutes at my best.

6 months down the line I weighed 74 kilos and 12 months down the line I was at 70. In around 13-14 months I had shed 10 kilos in all. Today I weigh around 66 kilos. But wait, weight loss was just a by-product for me. The real results are below:
- HbA1c in April 2015 – 9.8 – in the danger zone
- HbA1c in March 2016 – 6 – in the prediabetic zone

From a chronic diabetic my status changed to that of a prediabetic. Which means that I had really succeeded in fighting diabetes aggressively and in keeping my blood glucose within permissible levels. Which further means that I had pushed away (or escaped) the long term complications of diabetes like failed kidneys, blindness, heart problems and a stroke to name a few.

I keep oscillating between the gym and just walking in the open. But honestly, I am more regular when I just walk. Walking is a panacea for diabetes. It suits any weight (unless you have other medical issues that walking can worsen), any body type, any season, any time of the day. It provides us immense flexibility and great results. Yes, one does need to be patient and persistent and the results are bound to follow.

Cut to March of 2020 and the great pandemic. In the initial days there was a restriction on everything including walking in the open. A month went by without any form of exercise. And I was getting extremely scared of upsetting a beautifully balanced weight of 65 kilos and an HbA1c of 6. In those days I followed a lot of news and one of things getting covered regularly was about how people were exercising at home. Weight training, cardio, yoga, aerobics, everything was happening, at home. Physical classes for some of these went online and the committed lot continued to burn their calories.

Motivated by this I started doing 2 things:
- Walking at home
- Spot jogging at home

Now walking at home is very different from walking in an open space. My walking perimeter in the open is 1.5kms and the entire length of my hall is a few steps. Frustrating! But I had to continue walking. So I started distracting myself by having the music on or watching TV while I walked. It started making a lot of difference and I wasn't bored anymore. In fact I started lining up important interviews for consumption during my walk. Some old, some contemporary. Some topical and some documentaries. My walking time became extremely productive for me.

Now switching gears. When we walk in the open, simply because of the sheer amount of space we have, it becomes possible for us to walk for 50-60 minutes and even beyond at a go. When we walk at home, walking for an hour at a stretch is tough. Now this led to me walking in installments. Here is how it goes:

My total walk for the day is 8000 steps and it takes me 80 minutes. I simply split that by 3. Remember I started this just to kill my boredom with walking long durations at home, not with any other plan in mind.

- I walked for 2000 steps after breakfast (after a gap of 30 minutes after breakfast)
- I walked for 2000 steps before or after lunch (if before then the walk would be over at least 30 minutes before my lunch and if later then after a gap of 30 minutes)
- I walked for 4000 steps in the evening, say between 5pm and 6pm, and that at least 90 minutes before dinner

I settled into this routine very well. In the meantime the checking of my blood sugar levels on the glucometer resumed. Now my checking patterns are like this: I check regularly for a few days and then I don't maybe check for a month. And then I check again. The results on my glucometer screen surprised me. My postprandial readings (readings that we take 120 minutes from the time we start eating) were never above 150. In fact the maximum numbers of readings were in the range of 120 to 135. I never touched 160 ever in that period. My fasting reading, which would be in the range of 100 to 110, came down to between 90 and 100. And my HbA1c from 6 came down to a magical 5.8 in 6 months. All this happened between April and September 2020. I had never gone below 6 since 2014. After some time I started going down to very low sugar levels between meals, sometimes to as low as 70 and I had to increase my intake accordingly. This process led to a decrease in the daily dosage of metformin. It came down from 1350mg per day to 1000 mg. My doctor added 0.2mg of voglibose just to take care of my post meal levels. What happened after that is another story for me to tell in chapter 11.

Did you understand what happened? Let me decode it for you.

- Before the lockdown I would walk 60-80 minutes at one go.
- This helped me keep my sugar levels in check and be active in general. But the influence of that walk helped me with only that meal or time of day. Of course my overall glycaemic control was fantastic and I am not denying that.
- But with these intermittent walks thrice a day, what I did was (without being aware initially) influence my blood sugar levels after each meal or snack.
- If I walked before the meal or the snack, I would end up eating on a lower pre-meal or pre-snack blood sugar level, which in turn controlled the post-meal / post-snack spike.

  Example - Say I walked before lunch and at lunch my blood sugar level was 90. I then have 50 points to work with, given the fact that I am always aiming for tight control. And with the understanding about food that we have now, (owing to the previous chapter and the 14-day exercise in chapter 9), I will never go wrong.
- If I walked after the meal or the snack, I would work at neutralising its ability to increase my postprandial blood sugar levels.

  Example - Say I walked for 20 minutes after lunch. Without the walk, my sugar levels would have risen to say 160. But the 20 minute-walk helped me restrict that rise to 150.
- Finally, never underestimate the 5 or 10 points difference that you make after each meal. In glycaemic terms they mean a lot. When they add up like this, you will gain brilliant glycaemic control over a period of time and your next HbA1c may be a pleasant surprise for you. In my case at an HbA1c of 6 my average blood sugar level for the quarter was 125 and at an HbA1c of 5.8 it came down to 120.

You would have realised that I just used the words - **intermittent walking**. If you are familiar with the diabetes ecosystem you may have heard of terms like intermittent fasting. I have just showcased to you how intermittent walking can help you and how you can still have all your meals and snacks without limiting yourself to extreme diet forms. A walk is more sustainable than a fad. It is a strategic weapon.

The moral of the story is:

Burn some
calories and then eat
OR
Eat and then burn
some calories

Keep moving!

It is time to assess the walks that you have been taking and correspond them with the ultimate goal, your HbA1c. Is the result satisfactory? If not you may want to try this: assume you walk for 50 minutes a day at one stretch and that covers 5000 steps for you. Now sit back and decide how you would like to split these 50 minutes (5000 steps) over the day. There are a few factors that you need to consider.

- Am I just walking or am I also walking to compensate for those times of the day:
    - when I have a higher calorie intake
    - when for that part of the day, there is no medication or the dosage is much lesser
- What will suit me - a pre-meal walk or a post-meal walk
- And finally how do I fit this into my regular daily routine

A PRESCRIPTION WITH A DESCRIPTION...

06

...understand your medication

When we go to our medical professionals for regular one-off severe or not-so-severe illnesses or diseases, we know that the prescription given by our doctors will do their job. The medicines in the prescribed dosages will cure us within a certain time period. These are closed-ended and time-bound ailments. But when you have diabetes you have a medical condition for a lifetime. Please note that in the case of diabetes I have not used the word 'disease'. In my personal definition a disease or an illness is something which has a cure. Diabetes is a condition, similar to many other auto-immune conditions that simply have no cure and can only be managed. As we saw in chapter 2, the ominous octet makes it that much more complicated.

As a diabetic - a new diabetic, a not so-new diabetic, as someone who has lived with diabetes for very long (or as a caretaker), have you ever tried to understand the kind of medication/s your doctor has put you on? Have you understood why a certain class / classes of medications have been prescribed to you and not something else? Do you know why some medicines are taken before a meal and some after? Do you understand the difference between sustained release medications and those that regulate post-food hyperglycemia (increase in blood sugar levels)? I am sure that many of you haven't given this a second thought.

So here is my mega-question - don't you think that it is imperative and important for you to understand the nature of the medicines that you will be on for a life-time? In the case of one-off illnesses it seems ok to not have that curiosity. But in the case of diabetes knowing your medication can be an asset and aid you in good diabetes management. And that is exactly what the title of this chapter implies.

Before going ahead it becomes important for me to give you the physician's side of the story. Have you ever thought of what doctors consider or what are the factors they look at when they write our prescriptions down? Here is a small insight.

For the medical fraternity, glycaemic control (indicated by HbA1c) remains suboptimal despite the wide range of available medications. A more effective medication prescription might result in better control. However, the process by which physicians choose glucose-lowering medicines is poorly understood. The following is an excerpt from a research done amongst physicians (respondents). The respondents weighed the importance of 15 patient, physician, and nonclinical factors when deciding which medications to prescribe for type 2 diabetic subjects at each of three management stages.

Stage 1 is initiation. **Stage 2** is when the use of a second-in-line oral agent is prescribed. **Stage 3** is insulin therapy.

While there were differences in the outcomes of GPs and those of specialists, as an **overall there were five major considerations at each stage. The most frequently cited considerations included - overall assessment of the patient's health/comorbidity, A1C level, and**

patient's adherence behavior. For insulin initiation, some physicians placed greater emphasis on patient adherence. General practitioners also identified patient fear of injections and patient desire to prolong non-insulin therapy as major insulin barriers. But as summary, qualitative factors like adherence, motivation and overall health assessment were somewhat more highly considered than quantitative factors like A1C, age, weight etc.
Credit: https://care.diabetesjournals.org/content/30/6/1448

As a diabetic for 14 years and now as a certified diabetes educator, I understand this pharmacology well enough to take care of myself, in consultation with my doctor. I understand the reason for being on 500mg of Glycomet (metformin) SR 500 (1———1———X) and Vobit (voglibose) 0.2mg (1———X———1). I understand how these help me manage my day better and further allow me to give accurate feedback to my doctor about their effectiveness for my specific routine and lifestyle.

Now that you have understood the parameters your doctor uses to prescribe to you, allow me to explain to you the reasons for insisting on a 'prescription with a description':

1 Every class of medicine (in the diabetes context) serves a particular purpose in diabetes management. As a diabetic you need to know what medicine/s you are on and how it is helping you. Understanding the class / classes of medicines the doctor has prescribed to you will help you understand how the doctor has profiled you. **Quickly refer back to chapter 2 here and you will understand the correlation between the (ominous octet) 8 reasons for hyperglycemia and the medicine classes mentioned in the table that appears later in this chapter.**

    a.   This could go on to mean that you are a very compliant, moderately compliant or a non-compliant patient. Has your doctor been forced to increase your dosage or change the medication class to compensate for your non-adherence? Are you still in the habit of having refined foods and following an inactive and lethargic lifestyle? This includes parameters like your weight and your glycaemic control (HbA1c).

b. This could also indicate to you the stage of the diabetes life-cycle you are in. Is it Initiation or do you now need a second-in-line oral medicine or are you ready to start insulin therapy?. For example, it could be that you are a pre-diabetic and your doctor has put you on minimal medication as mere support. This is an initiation or a pre-initiation stage. Here there is a higher onus on you to ensure good glycaemic control through lifestyle changes and stop yourself from getting into the diabetes zone. When you answer these questions for yourself with the help of a discussion with your doctor, the following will happen.

2   Your next goal/s as far as your diabetes management goes will take shape. Here are a few examples of what you may understand, feel and decide accordingly:

a. "I do not like the fact that my doctor has added more medicines to the list. I should look at cutting down on my carbohydrate intake and adopt whole foods."

b. "During my next visit I want to go back to my old medication. I should start walking to achieve healthier blood sugar levels."

c. "I want to bring my HbA1c level back to 7 from the current 8.5. I have to refocus on diet and exercise to achieve this. I do not want my doctor to add more medicines to my list. I need to manage my work-related stress better."

d. "I want to lose 10 kilos in the next 8 months. I hope that this weight loss will help me cut down on the medicines and also make my body less insulin resistant. I should be able to manage my diabetes through a healthy diet and exercise with minimal help from medicines."

e.   "I do not want to start insulin. I am going to try my best to improve my glycaemic control by the end of this quarter."

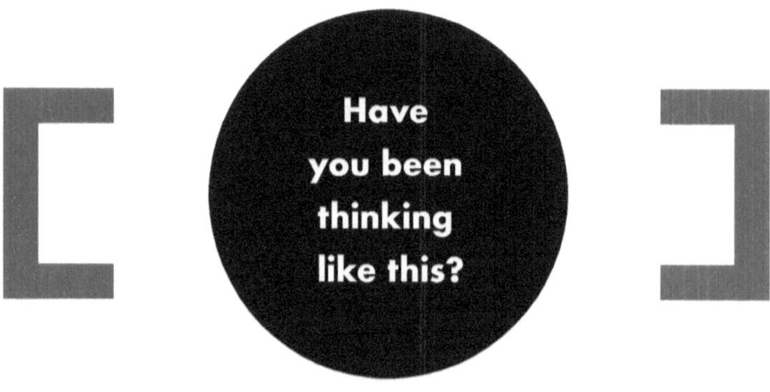

If not then you should begin to do so. Let me also tell you that with good glycaemic control, you will have the 'good-to-have-problems' knocking at your door. When your glycaemic control improves and stays that way for a sustained period of time, you will go through another small transient phase during which you and your doctor will again go through the process of finding a set of optimal medications for you. More of that in chapter 11.

Let us now understand the various classes of diabetes medications. They are:

OAD: Oral Antidiabetic Drugs

OHD: Oral Hypoglycemic Agents

Insulin preparation (Both Type 1 and Type 2 DM):
Short acting, Intermediate acting, Long acting, Analogues

The 'Action' part of the following table (column 3) is the one that corresponds to and aims to compensate for one or more of the 8 reasons (the ominous octet) that lead to high blood sugar levels.

Therapeutic Category	Drug Name/ Class	Action	Expected HbA1c reduction
Biguanide	Metformin	Reduce hepatic glucose production and decreased insulin resistance	0.5 - 0.8%
Sulphonylureas (Insulin Secretagogues)	Glimipride, Glilbenclamide, Gliclazide	Stimulate the beta cells to stimulate insulin secretion	1 - 2 %
Thiazolidinedione	Pioglitazone	Reduce insulin resistance in body tissues	0.5 - 1.4%
Alpha Glucose Inhibitor (AGI)	Acarbose, Voglibose	Reduce the absorption of carbohydrates from the intestine	1 - 2 %
Dipeptidyl Peptidase - 4 (DPP-4) Inhibitors	Vildagliptin, Sitagliptin, Saxagliptin Linagliptin	Reduce the degradation of incretins	0.5 - 1%
Glucagon-like peptide -1 (GLP-1) agonists	Exenatide inj., Liraglutide inj.	Stimulate the secretion of incretins	0.5 - 0.8%
Sodium-Glucose Co-transporter-2 (SGLT2) inhibitors	Canagliflozin, Dapagliflozin, Empagliflozin	Increase urinary glucose excretion	0.5 - 0.9%
Insulin	Short acting, Intermediate acting, Long acting, Analogues	Reduction of blood sugar levels	> 2%

Here is the exercise that you need to now do. Look up the medicines you are on and understand what purpose they serve in your body for your diabetes management. When you do this you will also understand the holistic nature of the treatment your doctor has designed for you especially with respect to the 8 reasons that can cause hyperglycemia.

CHAPTER EXERCISE

List your diabetes medications and write down what they do for you.

Brand Name	Class	Action

 Complete this before you move onto the next chapter.

DIALOGUES
WITH
YOURDOCT
OR...

DIALOGUES WITH YOUR DOCTOR...

07

...it's a two way street

Let me dedicate the first part of this chapter to our relationships with our doctors. Do we treat them as friends or as people who, if given a chance, we would never want to meet again? Why do some of us look forward to our quarterly doctor visits and why do some of us detest and prolong these meetings? Let us look at the various nuances of the patient-doctor relationship.

This quote sums up the patient's side of the story.

> **"The patient will never care how much you know, until they know how much you care."**

Keeping in line with the spirit of this quote let me outline the patient's perspective and expectation from his / her doctor.

- Patients want to be able to trust the competence and efficacy of their doctors.
- Patients want to be able to leverage the health care

system effectively.

- Patients want to be treated with dignity and respect.
- Patients want their doctors to be honest with them and help them understand how their sickness or treatment will affect their lives.
- Patients want to discuss the effect their illness will have on their family, friends, and finances.
- Patients worry about the future and they want their doctors to empathise with them.
- Patients worry about and want to learn how to care for themselves away from the clinical setting.
- Patients want physicians to focus on their pain, physical discomfort, and <u>functional disabilities.</u>

Another way of interpreting the above is as follows - if you are a type 2 diabetic and have all these concerns, then you are in the right direction with respect to your diabetes management. A patient who has these concerns is clearly someone who wants to get better and **be in control.**

And I agree with this whole approach. At least for most of the diseases that a doctor treats us for, and I am here referring to diseases that have a beginning and an end. But there are a different set of diseases or conditions that have a beginning, but no end. They may start at various stages of our lives, but they unfortunately stay with us till we are. Type 2 diabetes is one of them. Such diseases or conditions go onto create a part 2 in the above equation. Which clearly is the doctor's side of the story and his or her set of expectations from us, the patients. Below are the doctor's expectations from a patient who has type 2 diabetes:

- **Doctors want us to follow the prescribed medication and lifestyle related advice.**
- **Doctors want us to focus on weight management.**
- **Doctors want us to be regular for appointments.**
- **Doctors want us to monitor our blood sugar levels regularly.**
- **Doctors want us to understand the ill-effects**

of sustained hyperglycemia.

- Doctors:
    - get upset when we, while progressing well, suddenly adopt an alternative form of therapy or lifestyle without consultation
    - feel let down when we go back to them after a long gap or interval with heightened blood sugar levels and have to begin all over again
    - don't like it when we end up coming for an appointment without doing the prescribed tests. Frankly that's a waste of everybody's time and our money
- Doctors want us to provide real feedback and not lie
- Doctors would like us to get contextually smarter over a period of time

Here is something I wrote 3 years ago on my blog and it sums up all that we just spoke about very well.

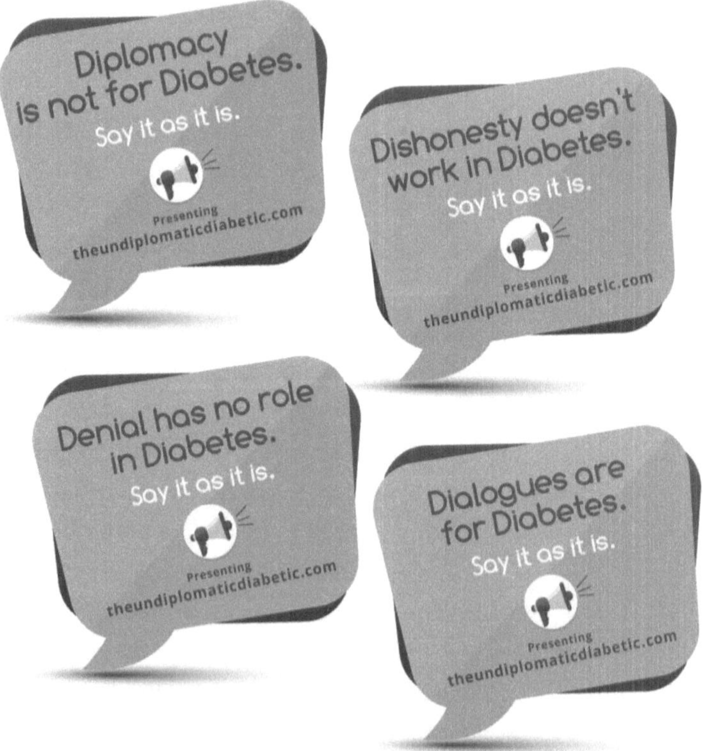

Now that we have set the context, you should also know that there already exist various relationship models for a patient-doctor relationship. I am just going to help you retrofit diabetes management into an overlap of two of these that I find the most relevant - the **'guidance-cooperation'** model and the **'mutual participation'** model.

The **'guidance-cooperation'** model comes into play at the beginning of the doctor-patient relationship. This would in most cases coincide with diagnosis, education and handholding at the early stages. The relationship evolves and moves into the **mutual participation** stage as the line of treatment is established, the patient is better educated about his or her condition, understands the negatives of an untreated and unmanaged diabetes and / or both the doctor and the patient work with regular monitoring, reports, opportunities and challenges to modify and optimise the treatment plan depending on the progression of type 2 diabetes in each patient. These models, as the names suggest, will work to their best only with patient participation.

While we want our doctors to cut across the dimensions of functionality and expression, we should also realise that adherence is the 'give' in the equation. The **"functional"** component involves the competence of the doctor in delivering the technical aspects of care such as: performing diagnostic tests, physical examinations and prescribing treatments. The **"expressive"** component reflects the art of medicine, including the affective portion of the interaction such as warmth and empathy, and how the doctor approaches the patient. **"Adherence"** from the patient is what makes the treatment effective. This simply means that the treatment is largely dependent on the patient carrying out the directions of the physician (i.e., compliance), like the ones I have listed in the doctor's expectations earlier.

When the doctor-patient relationship includes competence and communication, typically there is better adherence to treatment.

When better adherence to treatment is combined with patient satisfaction and care, improved health and better quality of life are the expected results.

. . . .

A critical 'functional' aspect of a patient-doctor relationship is when the doctor looks at your reports. When it comes to type 2 diabetes, there are many reports that your doctor may want to look at periodically. Apart from keeping tabs on your blood sugar levels they also go on to indicate the health of various organs in your body that may be affected due to long-lasting diabetes. Some tests may need to be done more often if you are not doing too well or not progressing as per your doctor's expectations. But if you are complying and tolerating the line of treatment, then with better results on the report card the frequency of these tests may decrease. Without these test results your doctor cannot prescribe an optimal line of treatment nor make any changes to the existing treatment plan. Stepping into your doctor's clinic without 'recent' reports is a waste of time and money.

Many of you may already know about the various complications that untreated and unmanaged diabetes can lead to. But the objective of this half of the chapter is not to educate you about the complications in isolation. The attempt is to help you see the **correlation between these complications and the tests** that you need to do to detect them early, or better, rule them out. If you detect them early enough you may be able to save one precious organ in your body from irreversible damage.

The reasons for my sharing this particular perspective with you are as follows. Over the last 6 years I have interacted socially with many family members, friends and colleagues who have type 2 diabetes. **Here is what I found out they don't know:**
- **Many of them, even in a city like Mumbai, do not know what an HbA1C test is**

- They do not know what sustained high blood sugars can do to their bodies, their minds and their families
- Given that they don't understand these complications, they do not know about any of the corresponding tests
- And unfortunately they become aware only when it is too late. A gangrene has set in or kidney damage has begun

I feel that tests prescribed in isolation or without a context are never usually followed-through by patients, unless the doctor is very persuasive. The same logic of a prescription (in this case a test) without a description applies here too. In some cases when the doctor gets tough, patients simply change their doctors. The only way out is education. Get type 2 diabetics to understand why these tests are important. So here we are:

The table on the next page summarises many of the tests that can be done to identify complications from diabetes, including those tests done during a physical examination. The physical examination evaluates your overall health. The doctor pays special attention to your eyes, blood vessels, heart, lungs, nerves, abdomen, and feet.

Organ or condition	Test	What it shows
High blood sugar	Every 3 to 6 months, have a hemoglobin A1c test.	How steady your blood sugar levels have been over time
High blood pressure	Have your blood pressure checked once at least a year. If your blood pressure is high, have it checked more often.	Pressure of blood flow in your arteries
Kidneys	Every year, have your urine checked for the protein albumin. Also, have your blood checked for the waste product creatinine. These are used to calculate an estimated glomerular filtration rate (eGFR).	Whether kidney disease is developing
Eyes	Every year, visit an ophthalmologist or an optometrist for a dilated eye examination (ophthalmoscopy). Some doctors may recommend less frequent eye examinations (for example, every 2 years) if you have no signs of diabetic retinopathy.	Whether retinopathy (damage to back of the eye) has developed
Feet	Every year, get a thorough examination of your feet.	Whether foot ulcers have developed Whether the person has lost any sensation
Teeth	Your dentist will recommend how often to have routine checkups. Many people should see their dentists once or twice a year.	Gum disease
Liver	Your doctor may recommend a liver function blood test, especially if you are taking a medicine that could affect your liver.	Liver disease
High cholesterol	Every year get your cholesterol levels checked.	Along with other measures, cholesterol levels can help you know your risk for heart attack or stroke

Treat this table as an overview.
This is just to get started off.

People like us with type 2 diabetes are at risk for long-term problems affecting the eyes, kidneys, heart, brain, feet, and nerves. The best way to prevent or delay these problems is to control our blood sugar and take good care of ourselves. Here are some more details.

Eyes

It is recommended that people with diabetes see an eye doctor every year for a dilated eye exam. Eye problems that can occur with diabetes include:

- Cataracts: A clouding of the lens of the eyes
- Glaucoma: Increased pressure in the eye
- Retinopathy: Eye changes with the retina in the back of the eye

Symptoms of eye problems include

- They can be asymptomatic in some cases
- Blurred vision
- Spots or lines in your vision
- Watery eyes
- Eye discomfort
- Loss of vision

Kidneys

Have your urine checked for protein at least once a year. Protein in the urine is a sign of kidney disease. High blood pressure might also lead to kidney disease. Your blood pressure should be checked when you see your healthcare provider. Symptoms of a kidney problem include:

- Swelling of the hands, feet, and face
- Weight gain from edema
- Itching and/or drowsiness.
  (This can occur with end stage kidney disease.)

Heart and brain ·

All people with diabetes have an increased chance for heart disease and strokes. Heart disease is the major cause of death in people with diabetes. It is important to control other risks such as high blood pressure and high fats (cholesterol), as well as blood sugar.

<u>Symptoms of a heart attack include:</u>
- Shortness of breath
- Feeling faint
- Feeling dizzy
- Sweating
- Nausea
- Chest pain or pressure
- Pain in the shoulders, jaw, and left arm

<u>Warning signs of a stroke include:</u>
- Sudden numbness or weakness in the face, arm, or leg, usually on one side of the body.
- Sudden nausea
- Fever
- Vomiting
- Difficulty speaking or understanding words or simple sentences
- Sudden blurred vision or decreased vision in one or both eyes
- Difficulty swallowing
- Dizziness
- Loss of balance or loss of coordination
- Brief loss of consciousness
- Sudden inability to move part of the body (paralysis)
- Sudden intense headache

Feet ·

High blood sugars can lead to poor blood flow and nerve damage. This can lead to slow healing of sores. You can experience severe pain, but you can also lose feeling in your feet. In serious cases, this may lead to amputation of your toes, foot, or leg.

Nerves

High blood sugars can affect all of the nerve endings in your body. Nerve damage can cause many problems. Symptoms of nerve damage include:

- Burning pain
- Numbness
- Tingling or loss of feeling in the feet or lower legs
- Constipation and diarrhea
- Problems with sexual function in both men and women

Neuropathy

Neuropathy is a disorder of the nervous system that can affect people with diabetes. There are different forms of neuropathy, including:

- Peripheral neuropathy: Damage to the peripheral nervous system
- Autonomic Type I: Damage to the nerves of internal organs
- Gastroparesis: Movement of food through the stomach slows or stops
- Postural hypotension: Drop in blood pressure due to change in body position
- Uncontrolled diarrhea

I sincerely hope that you are starting to appreciate the reasons for these tests, quarter after quarter, once in six months or annually.

While all the above are the bodily complications of unmanaged type 2 diabetes, lets us not forget our minds. Depression is another diabetes complication. Here is something that I had written a few years back. It addresses the non-diabetics in the society and the sensitivity they need to have with respect to their diabetic family member, friend or colleague. I think it aptly describes the vicious cycle that depression can get a diabetic into.

Once a diabetic, always a diabetic. Easier said than done. Unlike someone like you who has the fortune of good health, a diabetic is forced to live a million lifetimes in one. Stress, frustration, anger, hopelessness and an entire bouquet of negative emotions can invade a person with diabetes over a period of time.

While this feeling can be devastating for a diabetic, YOU as a family member, a friend or a colleague while wanting to help can completely miss the point and lack empathy. Here are a few things that you can learn about for your diabetic:
When a person you know has diabetes, whether newly diagnosed or a longstanding one, living with it can be overburdening to say the least. Some of the emotions they will periodically go through can include: Grief, Anxiety, Bitterness, Disappointment and Stress.

If someone you care for has diabetes, it is important for you to know that they are prone to depression 3 times more than someone without it. Research has found that people who suffer from both diabetes and depression have poorer metabolic and glycaemic control which has, in turn, been found to intensify symptoms of depression. Depression can affect a patient's capacity to deal with their diabetes, including managing blood glucose levels appropriately.

Such people are further at greater risk of suffering from an episode of diabetic burnout which collectively can have adverse effects on physical health and potentially instigate more long term complications both to do with diabetes and independent of it. Depressed people with diabetes are less likely to adhere to medication and diet regimens and subsequently have a reduction in quality of life and increased health care expenditure.

Diabetes is overwhelming. It is important to recognise that this could be happening to someone you care for. Be kind and remember to redirect your diabetic to professional help. A doctor can help treat depression. By helping address depression you are helping your loved one, a friend or a colleague to achieve better glycaemic control, a positive state-of-mind and a significantly improved quality of life.

THINGS
YOU MAY
NEVER ASK
YOUR
DOCTOR...

THINGS YOU MAY NEVER ASK YOUR DOCTOR...

08

...did you know about the dawn phenomenon?

At this stage, you know quite a bit about diabetes management. You have learnt all that you have needed to learn about food, exercise and medication. You have understood the complications that a badly managed diabetes can lead to. You have also understood the tests that you need to do on a periodic basis to ensure regular screening to be able to detect the start of any complication early enough to not let it deteriorate any further.

Let me now talk to you about 4 things that may not come up during your conversations with your doctor. In my case it came up because my mother asked the doctor. I had no clue earlier that a symptom like snoring could be related to type 2 diabetes. I think it is important for you to know about these as they may, in certain scenarios, become critical to your effort and potential results.

Three out of these (dawn phenomenon, somogyi effect and obstructive sleep apnea) come in the way of good diabetes management and the fourth one (time-in-range) helps you take your diabetes management a notch higher.

Let's now get to them one by one.

1 and 2. **Dawn phenomenon and Somogyi effect**

I am bracketing both of them together here because while the causes are different, the result they produce is the same - **high sugar levels in the mornings.** The dawn phenomenon happens naturally, but the somogyi effect usually happens because of problems with your diabetes management routine.

You already know that your body uses a form of sugar called glucose as its main source of energy. The hormone insulin, which your pancreas makes, helps your body move glucose from your bloodstream to your cells. While you sleep, your body doesn't need as much energy. But when you're about to wake up, it gets ready to burn more fuel. It tells your liver to start releasing more glucose into your blood. That should ideally trigger your body to release more insulin to handle more blood sugar. But when you have diabetes, your body doesn't make enough insulin to do that. That leaves too much sugar in your blood, a problem called hyperglycemia. And sustained high blood sugars, as we have just seen can result in irreversible health problems.

This is how the the dawn phenomenon and the somogyi effect are different:

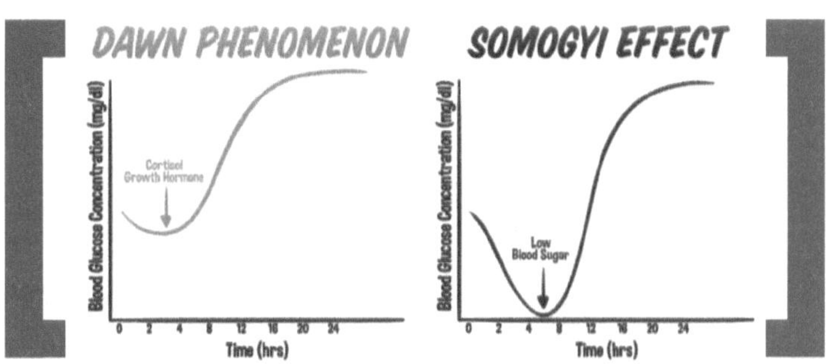

The Dawn Phenomenon . . . .

If you have diabetes, your body doesn't release more insulin to match the early-morning rise in blood sugar. This is called the dawn phenomenon, since it usually happens between 3 a.m. and 8 a.m. The dawn phenomenon happens to nearly everyone with diabetes. But there are a few ways to prevent it, including:

- Not eating carbohydrates before going to bed.
- Changing the time / dosage of your diabetes medication or insulin at night.
- Using an insulin pump overnight.

You can make these changes in consultation with your doctor.

The Somogyi Effect . . . .

The Somogyi effect also causes high levels of blood sugar in the early morning. But it usually happens when you take too much or too little insulin before bed, or when you skip your nighttime snack. When that happens, your blood sugar can drop sharply overnight. Your body responds by releasing hormones that work against insulin. That means you'll have too much blood sugar in the morning. This is also called rebound hyperglycemia.

How do you know which one you have?

Your doctor will want to find out why you're waking up with high blood sugar before they tell you how to treat it. This means they'll ask you to test your blood sugar in the middle of the night – around 2 or 3 a.m. — for several nights.

If your levels are always low during that time, it's probably the somogyi effect. If not, it's likely the dawn phenomenon. Knowing which is which will help your doctor come up with a plan to address it.

3. Obstructive Sleep Apnea (OSA) . . . .

Snoring can make for a bad night's sleep. But if it happens because you have obstructive sleep apnea (OSA), it's a sign of a bigger problem. The condition raises your risk for other health issues like high blood pressure and diabetes. But when you treat sleep apnea, you can ease or even cure some of these issues. Here are some health problems (not exhaustive) that you may face if you have sleep apnea:

High blood pressure - If you already have it, sleep apnea can make it worse. When you wake up often during the night, your body gets stressed. That makes your hormone systems go into overdrive, which boosts your blood pressure levels. Also, the level of oxygen in your blood drops when you can't breathe well, which may add to the problem.

Treatment can make a difference, though. Some people with high BP who get help for sleep apnea will see their blood pressure improve. Their doctors may be able to cut back on their BP medications. But you shouldn't stop or change your dose without talking to your doctor first.

Heart disease - People with OSA are more likely to have heart attacks. The cause may be low oxygen. Strokes and atrial fibrillation – a fast, fluttering heartbeat – are also linked with the condition. Sleep apnea disrupts how your body takes in oxygen, which makes it hard for your brain to control how blood flows in your arteries and the brain itself.

Type 2 diabetes - Sleep apnea is common among people with this condition – 80% or more of them may have OSA. Obesity raises a person's risk for both disorders. Although studies haven't shown a cause-and-effect link between sleep apnea and type 2 diabetes, not getting enough shut-eye can keep your body from using insulin properly, which leads to diabetes.

In my own case, my doctor advised me to use a CPAP (continuous positive airway pressure machine). Instead, I decided to lose weight. My OSA has vanished and I know I have helped myself in my diabetes management by doing that.

Weight gain - Extra weight raises your chances of getting sleep apnea, and the condition also makes it harder to slim down. When you're overweight, you can have fatty deposits in your neck that block breathing at night. On the flip side, sleep apnea can make your body release more of the hormone ghrelin, which makes you crave carbs and sweets. And when you're tired all the time, you might not be able to turn the food you eat into energy as efficiently, which can lead to weight gain and increase your chance of developing type 2 diabetes.

Treatment for OSA can make you feel better, with more energy for exercise and other activities. This can help you lose weight, which can help your sleep apnea.

Time in range (TIR) . . . .

"Time-in-Range" (TIR) is the percentage of time that a person spends with their blood glucose levels in a target range. The range will vary depending on the person, but general guidelines suggest starting with a range of 70 to 180 mg/dl. (Over time, some people decide to aim for a tighter range, such as 70 to 140 mg/dl.)

In a single number, time-in-range captures a lot about how blood glucose levels might vary throughout a day or over time. The example graphics below show various levels of time-in-range, from 0% to 100%:

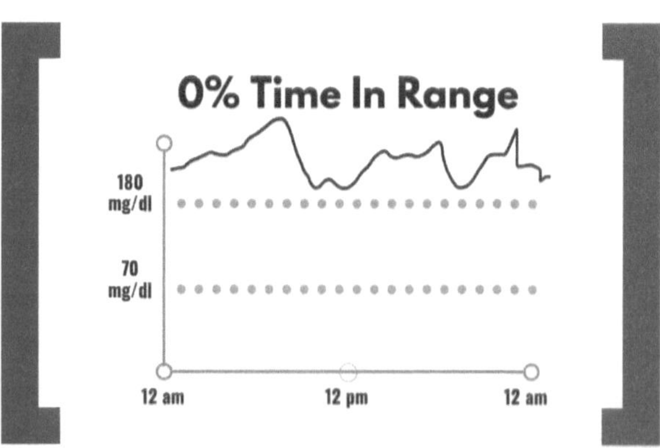

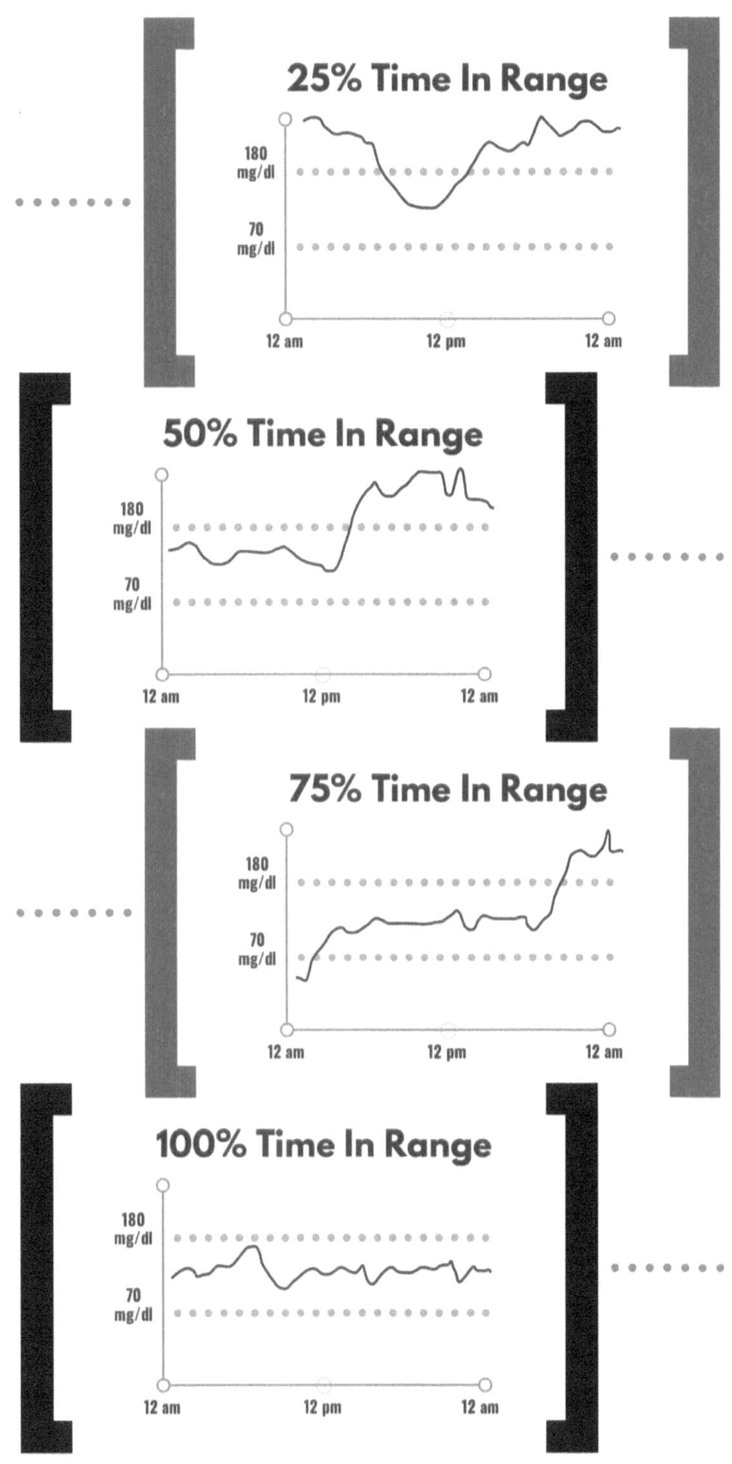

25% Time In Range
180 mg/dl
70 mg/dl
12 am
12 pm
12 am
50% Time In Range
180 mg/dl
70 mg/dl
12 am
12 pm
12 am
75% Time In Range
180 mg/dl
70 mg/dl
12 am
12 pm
12 am
100% Time In Range
180 mg/dl
70 mg/dl
12 am
12 pm
12 am

Time-in-range can also be understood as "hours per day" spent in-range. For example, 50% time-in-range (70-180 mg/dl) means 12 hours per day spent in-range.

Why is Time-in-Range Important?

TIR goes beyond A1C in representing blood glucose levels because it captures variation – the highs, lows, and in-range values that characterise life with diabetes. By contrast, A1C is a measure of average blood sugar over a two-to-three-month period; it cannot capture time spent in various blood glucose ranges. To illustrate the limitations of A1C and the advantages of time-in-range, see the graphics below. These three examples show three different people – all with the same average blood glucose (154 mg/dl) and the same A1C (7%). However, the highs, lows, and in-range blood glucose values are markedly different: the first person has a rollercoaster of dangerous highs and lows, the second has moderate variability and fewer highs and lows, and the third person has little variability with all time spent in-range.

People living with diabetes experience different energy levels, moods, and overall quality of life when they are "in-range" vs. "out-of-range." Time-in-range can capture these differences in a way A1C cannot.

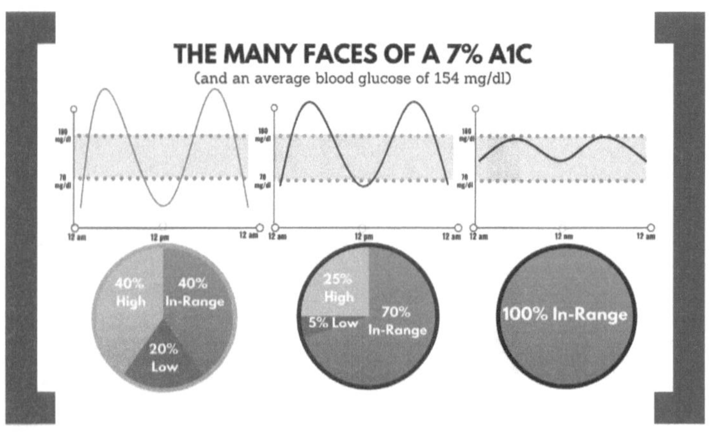

Because time-in-range can be measured at home (using a continuous glucose monitoring device) on a daily basis or weekly basis, it has a huge advantage over A1C and helps in understanding what behaviours and choices prompt more time-in-range, what drives blood glucose out-of-range, and where/when changes can be made (e.g., time of day). Thinking about blood glucose in terms of time-in-range offers a more nuanced, cause-and-effect understanding of diabetes than A1C. For instance, how do different foods affect your time-in-range? How does walking after meals affect your time-in-range? A1C cannot reveal these relationships.

I would sum-up time-in-range as a fine-tuned or a refined version of HbA1C. It adds a beautiful layer of limitation to it. In simple terms it tells us that simply achieving a good HbA1C is not enough. How you do it makes all the difference. Once you evolve your thinking to achieving good glycaemic control in the right manner, you will adopt time-in-range as your benchmark. This will automatically take your diabetes-management efforts to the highest level possible.

THE
FIRST 14
DAYS....

THE FIRST 14 DAYS...

... the ultimate short-cut

If you go back to the cover page of the book you will see the words - 'The ultimate short-cut to diabetes management' written on it. Maybe that was one of the reasons you picked this book up. Everybody who has type 2 diabetes is looking for a short-cut, an easy way to manage their diabetes. I did too. But here is the story of how I discovered it.

In the last quarter of 2013 my HbA1c reached an alarming 10. This meant that my average blood sugar level for that quarter was a dangerous 240. Fortunately or unfortunately at that time I was also in an organization that was taking my career nowhere. With my HbA1c as the final trigger I decided to quit my job. I started spending large amounts of time at home and simultaneously thinking about starting a new phase of my life, as far as my diabetes management went. I am an ardent tennis fan and had gathered quite a few autobiographies and books written by tennis greats. This sabbatical seemed a good time to catch up on all those books. One of the books that I had picked up was by Novak Djokovic, called 'serve to win'. I opened this book thinking that it would be one more autobiography. But when I started going through its contents I realised that the book was about the 'serving on a plate' and how that 'serving on a plate' could dictate the way someone's game changed on the tennis court.

To cut the long story short... Novak Djokovic is gluten-intolerant. He was once a player plagued by aches, breathing difficulties and injuries on court, thanks to a gluten-heavy diet. From that phase of his life to the year 2011 where he won a breathtaking 10 titles, three grand slams and forty three consecutive matches, Novak's journey is an inspiration. To achieve this Novak spent 14 days without gluten under Dr. Cetojevic's guidance. As he describes in his book, for the first week he craved for the comfort he found in those foods. But as the days rolled past, he began to feel different. He felt lighter and more energetic. The nighttime stuffiness he had lived with for fifteen years had suddenly disappeared. He no longer wanted those breads, rolls and cookies. Gluten was the sure-shot culprit that was pulling his body down and not allowing him to achieve physical and mental excellence.

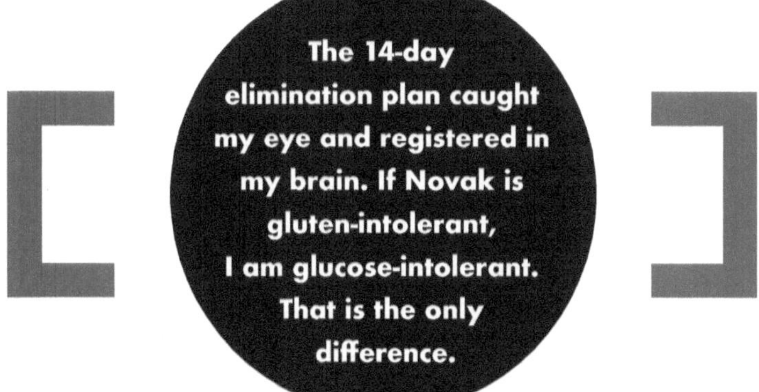

I decided to do the 14 day test myself, but a little differently. I executed this plan and after 140 blood sugar readings over 14 days (10 readings per day (over 5 meals) x 14 days), I knew what was good for me and what wasn't. I knew how much I could eat and I knew the limit my body was telling me to set for myself. Below is an illustration for one day.

Day 1 of 14 - 10 readings per day

Pre-meal reading	Pre-snack reading	Pre-meal reading	Pre-snack reading	Pre-meal reading
Breakfast (Details of what I had for breakfast)	**Mid-morning snack** (Details of what I had as a mid-morning snack)	**Lunch** (Details of what I had for lunch)	**Evening Snack** (Details of what I had as an evening snack)	**Dinner** (Details of what I had for dinner)
Items + portion sizes	Items + portion sizes	Items + portion sizes	Items + portion sizes	Items + portion sizes
Post-meal reading	Post-snack reading	Post-meal reading	Post-snack reading	Post-meal reading

Here's how you should go about it:

1. Vary every meal as much as possible.
2. Try out as many grains, dals, vegetables and fruits as possible. If you are a non-vegetarian try out everything that you would normally eat.
3. By the end of week one you will have: 7 days x 10 readings per day = 70 readings
4. You can use week 2 to test out more food variations or to adjust the portion sizes from week one. Let me explain both.
5. Food variations - You may realise that when you have rotis with potatoes, your postprandial sugar levels go up to 180, but when you replace potatoes with cauliflower or cabbage your postprandial readings go up to only 160. That's something learnt about potatoes and starchy vegetables.
6. Portion adjustment - Let's take the same example as above. When you have 4 rotis with cauliflower or cabbage your postprandial reading may go up to 160. But instead of 4 rotis if you have 3 and add a bowl of curd instead to fill your stomach with, your postprandial reading may go up to only 150. That's something learnt about cutting down on carbs

and substituting it with low glycaemic index foods to help
you feel full.

7. The pre-meal / pre-snack readings are critical because they
   help you understand when to eat your next meal or snack.
   When your pre-meal level is already 130, you will want to
   optimise your next meal to something lighter or do with a
   smaller portion and follow it up with a 20 minute walk. But
   when your pre-meal level is say just 100, you can take some
   liberties with your next meal.

8. **Now you have a hold on:**
   a. **What to eat**
   b. **How much to eat and**
   c. **When to eat**

9. Now extrapolate this logic. These are the permutations
   and combinations that you need to test for in these 14
   transformational days.

What do you achieve in these 14 days:

What you get by the end of these 14 days is a set of rules to follow.
A set of rules that include what you should eat and what you should
stay away from. A set of rules that tell you your thresholds in terms
of portion sizes. And most importantly a set of rules that you have
made for yourself. As a practice, you should repeat this exercise
whenever you encounter something new. For example when you
step out to eat and decide to have pani-puri, gol-gappa or puchka,
you need to realize that it is the meetha pani (the sweet water) that
upsets the cart. Otherwise the 6 puris with moong or boondi with the
khara pani (the spicy water) may be a perfect snack to have along
with an evening walk. **Dissect everything you eat in your
head first and then let your glucometer do the rest.**

So here is how your 14 week chart looks like. Go ahead and fill in
the blanks. Don't think of the next 13 days in advance. It may seem
daunting. Plan your meals and snacks in advance so that you don't
miss a single meal or day and take one day at a time.

CHA
PTER
EXER
CISE

CHAPTER EXERCISE

Create your own 14-day chart.

Day 1 Your Name: Month and Year:					
	Breakfast	**Mid-morning**	**Lunch**	**Evening**	**Dinner**
Pre-meal/ snack reading					
Details of the meal/ snack					
Post-meal/ snack reading					

Day 2	Your Name: Month and Year:				
	Breakfast	**Mid-morning**	**Lunch**	**Evening**	**Dinner**
Pre-meal/ snack reading					
Details of the meal/ snack					
Post-meal/ snack reading					

And so on until day 14.

Go about this exercise as if your life depends on it. It really does. And if you are enjoying it and discovering new things along the way and adding to your 'diabetes quotient', you may want to continue till day 21. I am sure that most of us would exhaust the variations we have in terms of the regular foods we normally eat with over 21 x 10 = 210 meal / snack variations.

Finally, the fact that I picked up Novak's book as my first read during the initial days of my sabbatical is what I call 'Good Luck'. I hope that this chapter does the same for you. It may be a good idea to start this exercise as you read the next few chapters in this book. The perspective is extremely important.

YOUR JOURNEY FROM 10 TO 7...

10

...calibrate your success

You may find parts of this chapter an antithesis to the previous one. This is because in real-life terms there will be a time-lapse of a couple years between when these two experiences would come true for you. I say two years or so as an average. You could achieve this level of understanding even within 6 months if you make good diabetes management your mainstay henceforth.

As you start reading this chapter, I hope you have finished your 14-day exercise or are in the process of doing it. It is important that you appreciate for yourself the benefits of these 14 days to understand what I am going to say next. I am sure by this time you have realised the importance of checking. It has told you so much and you are now in a readjustment mode. You are in the process of fine tuning all those aspects of your life that influence your blood sugar levels. Before I get into the calibration story, which is what this chapter is about, I would like to share a small personal experience with you. I call it - **Mind, Body and the Glucometer.**

Over the last 7 years my HbA1c has oscillated largely between 5.8 and 6.6. It has also been 7 years since I did my 14-day exercise. During this period my glucometer was my best friend. But over the last few years I haven't checked so much. This was another experiment I undertook to understand the level of conditioning I had achieved. Here is what I mean:

- I stopped checking to understand if I would be able to sustain healthy sugar levels even if I did not check after every meal.
- I stopped checking to understand if I would still know what to eat, how much to eat and when to eat without checking so frequently.
- I stopped checking to understand if there would be a void. A feeling of helplessness, a fear of having eaten something wrong. Of having eaten too early or too late. Of having eaten too less or too much.

I didn't want my glucometer to become a crutch without which I simply couldn't walk, in this case 'eat'.

Why did I do this experiment:

Motivation 1 - I was trying to shake off the overdependence on the glucometer. And that sure was setting in. This will happen to you too if you are going to get very particular about your blood sugar levels. I would say it is a good overdependence to have for a limited period of time.

Motivation 2 - The strips are costly. Take INR 25 as the average price for one branded strip available in India. Even if I did save one prick a day over 90 days, I would save INR 2250 in a quarter. Do the math. INR 9000 every year. When I check, I check at least 5 times a day. Now do the math again. Self-monitoring can sometimes be mindless and one needs to at some level rationalise this habit.

What do I keep constant when I stop checking for some time:

- My diet
- My exercise patterns
- My sleep patterns
- My stress levels (as much as possible)

What am I trying to tell you:

If you are largely in control with in-range HbA1c levels over 4-5 quarters at a go, then start applying your mind to what you are doing right. Make a mental check-list of the routine that is working so well for you and do not allow for too much variance in it. Once you are able to achieve this, you will gradually be able to second guess the glucometer and will need to cross-check only when the rhythm is broken, a medication or dosage is changed or during a transition period. I will explain what transitions mean in this context in chapter 11.

My glucometer is still my best friend, but the heightening of my diabetes-quotient and one prick less were both a very welcome phenomena.

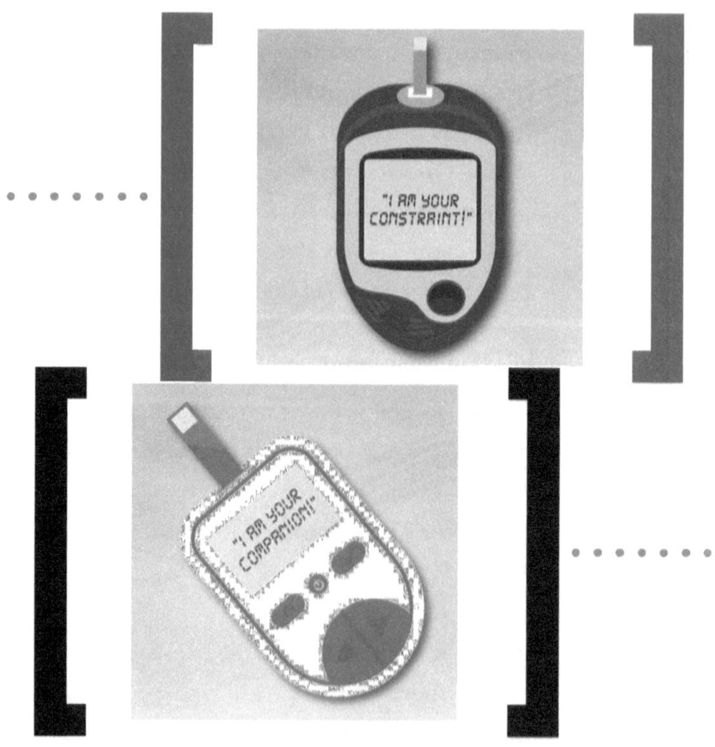

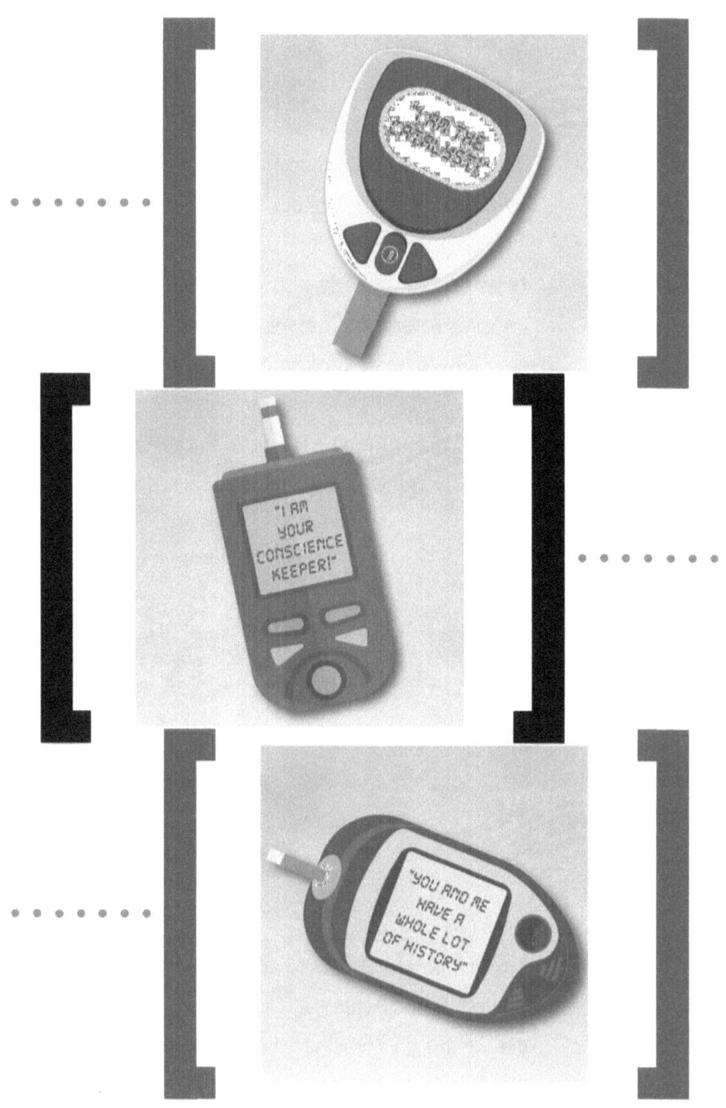

**These 5 images sum-up my relationship
with my glucometer.**

I hope you are getting the flow. Also please do not misunderstand the words 'stop checking'. This too is an interim phenomenon. **'For some time'** is the qualifier here, because my body has maintained a status quo and is responding well to the 3 critical variables (medication, food and exercise) and I intuitively know what my blood sugar levels will be. And hence I do not need to check so often. So in this situation of a status quo when do you check? Check to surprise yourself, check when you haven't planned to, check when you eat something new. But check once in a way, not so often.

Now this really was part one of the 'calibration' that the title of this chapter refers to. The second and the one that is equally important is what we have spoken about earlier in chapter 7. In chapter 7 we spoke about HbA1c as a measure of our glycaemic control and as one of the many test results that our doctor looks at. Let us now understand HbA1c in a little more detail.

HbA1c is referred to as the gold standard in monitoring glycaemic control in patients with diabetes. Since the beginning of clinical use in the 1970s, A1c has become an important tool. The role of the A1c test was broadened in 2010, when the American Diabetes Association (ADA) added A1c as a diagnostic criterion for diabetes and an A1c of > or = 6.5% was decided as a diagnostic criterion for diabetes, allowing the test to be used for the both diagnosis and management of diabetes. Recommending A1c as a diagnostic test was partly based on its advantages over timed glucose tests and the fact that it serves as a better index of overall glycaemic exposure and risk for long-term diabetes complications. It also does not require fasting or timed samples and becomes clinically more convenient.

The term HbA1c means glycated haemoglobin. It develops when haemoglobin, a protein within the red blood cells that carries oxygen throughout your body joins with the glucose in the blood becoming 'glycated'. By measuring glycated haemoglobin, doctors are able to get an overview of what our average blood sugar levels have been over a period of time. For people with diabetes, this is important as a relatively higher HbA1c indicates a greater risk of developing diabetes-related complications. We have looked at most diabetes-related complications and the tests thereof in chapter 7.

How does this work and why are we asked to measure our A1cs after every quarter

When our body processes sugar, glucose in the bloodstream naturally attaches to haemoglobin. The amount of glucose that attaches itself to this protein is directly proportional to the amount of sugar in your system at that time. Now our red blood cells last 8-12 weeks in our bodies before renewal and that is why an HbA1c reading is used to reflect the average blood glucose levels over that duration. From the time the red blood cells generate till the time they renew. Thereby providing a much more useful (in comparison to individual readings) measure to gauge a person's blood glucose control.

The accepted A1c calibrations are as follows:

- Less than 5.7% - No indication of diabetes
- 5.7% to 6.4% - Indication of prediabetes
- 6.5% or higher - Indication of diabetes

We have also, in one of the earlier chapters of this book, seen the staging model that corresponds to A1c levels and the progression of diabetes. Ideally people with diabetes should check results once every quarter. For uncontrolled diabetes the test should be done more frequently until agreed upon A1c goals are met.

Here is a ready reference of average blood sugars and their correspondence to A1c numbers:

If your A1c is 12.0%: Your average mean daily plasma blood sugar is around this (mg/dl): 298
If your A1c is 11.0%: Your average mean daily plasma blood sugar is around this (mg/dl): 269
If your A1c is 10.0%: Your average mean daily plasma blood sugar is around this (mg/dl): 240
If your A1c is 9.0%: Your average mean daily plasma blood sugar is around this (mg/dl): 212
If your A1c is 8.0%: Your average mean daily plasma blood sugar is around this (mg/dl): 183
If your A1c is 7.0%: Your average mean daily plasma blood sugar is around this (mg/dl): 154
If your A1c is 6.0%: Your average mean daily plasma blood sugar is around this (mg/dl): 126
If your A1c is 5.0%: Your average mean daily plasma blood sugar is around this (mg/dl): 97

As you internalise HbA1c and make it your benchmark for blood sugar control, don't forget to gradually take into consideration **time-in-range.** We have seen a detailed explanation of this in chapter 8. What I would like to add here from what I have read is as follows:

On a longer time horizon, early studies suggest time-in-range is just as good a predictor of long-term diabetes complications. Researchers found a strong relationship between different levels of time-in-range and diabetes complications: eye disease (retinopathy) and kidney disease (microalbuminuria). As time-in-range increased, complications decreased. Which when translated for patients like you and me means, tighter control to keep diabetes complications away.

Infact let's understand how 'time-in-range' looks for a non-diabetic.

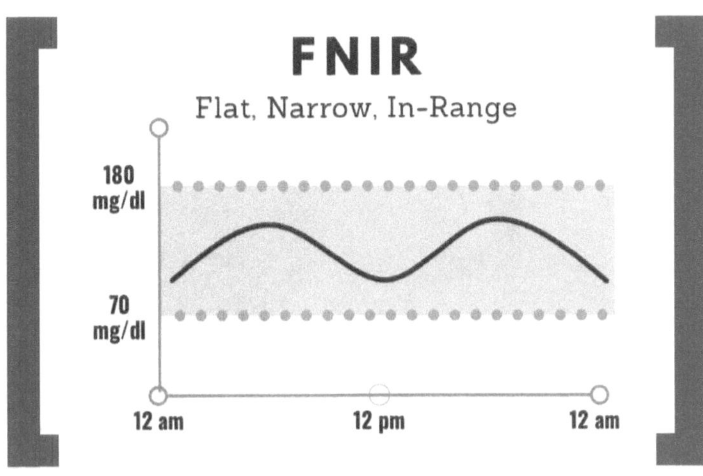

A recent study put continuous glucose (monitoring) meter (CGM) on people without diabetes for 10 days, finding 97% time-in-tight-range **(70-140 mg/dl)**, with blood glucose levels averaging 99 mg/dl and showing little variation. Consistent, in-range blood glucose levels are sometimes called <u>"flat, narrow, in-range"</u> (FNIR). This is one way to think about "ideal" blood sugars: **high time-in-range and flat glucose levels with few ups and downs. People with type 2 diabetes can strive for FNIR. On a day with FNIR levels, ask: What made that possible? How can I have more days like that?**

To determine your 'time-in-range, you should use at least 14 days' worth of blood glucose data. Time-in-range is most accurately measured using a continuous glucose meter (CGM), although a blood glucose meter (BGM) can also be used. You can speak to your doctor about this and then go ahead and take your diabetes management to the next level.

Diabetes - An individual sport

Once you have diabetes, you have your own number-game to play for the rest of your life. You have been diagnosed as a diabetic or a prediabetic because you fell under one of the criteria shown earlier. As a solo player your entire effort has to go towards keeping your readings within the allowable range. And all this for one reason – to live a healthy and a complication-free life.

As someone playing the diabetes game, you may be lucky enough to be able to afford a support system to anchor you. You may have the best diabetologist, nutritionist, chef, physical trainer and a life-coach by your side most of the time guiding you and helping you do things right. But there will be those zillion crucial moments every single day where you will be all alone to decide between the right and the wrong. And in those moments it will be your diabetes quotient, your level of awareness, your mental strength and your deliberate discretions that will decide whether you serve an ace or double fault. The spotlight is squarely on you.

CHAPTER EXERCISE

In the diabetes context, match the following from what we have learnt so far:

	My HbA1c is		I am
1.	6.5	A.	I am in the prediabetes stage
2.	5.8	B.	I am a diabetic and the probability of diabetes-complications having set in are also high
3.	9	C.	I am at the beginning of prediabetes stage
4.	5.7	D.	I am a non-diabetic
5.	5.1	E.	I am a diabetic

Answers: 1-E, 2-A, 3-B, 4-C, 5-D

TRANSIT
IONS
AND
TRANSF
ORMATI
ONS...

TRANSITIONS AND TRANSFORMATIONS...

11

... for the better or for the worse

Before starting to write this chapter let me tell what this is not about. This chapter is not about the stages in a diabetes lifecycle that takes into consideration merely one point - progression. If that is a constant then why should we all strive so much?

This chapter focusses on the various changes that you may go through as years go by. The main parameter that will affect all other variables is your HbA1c along with time-in-range. When that changes, your treatment plan will change. Of course all the other tests we have spoken about also hold true. I thought the best way to go through this chapter is to tell you my own story. Not in an emotional manner, but in a very objective and technical manner. So let's begin.

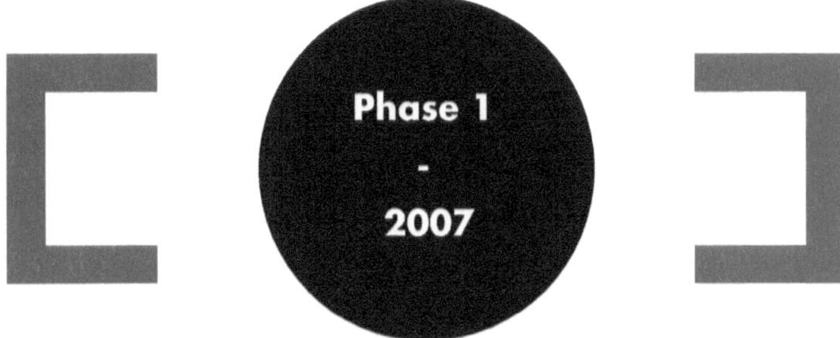

I was diagnosed with diabetes in 2007. I am sure I had it for much longer. It got diagnosed after a severe vertigo attack at work. I was in bed for 10 days and it used to take me 30 minutes to get up to go and use the bathroom. Post that some tests followed and I was declared a type 2 diabetic. I was only 36 years old then. My family doctor put me on Gluformin and Glimer and that is how my blood sugars got under some manageable levels. Here's the immediate month for you:

Date	Fasting reading	Postprandial reading
10th March 2007	305	Not taken
13th March 2007	279	327
24th March 2007	136	178
30th March 2007	118	178
2nd April 2007	107	Not taken
6th April 2007	105	130

I purchased my first glucometer in April 2007. I got it through an employee discount scheme for Rs.2100. It is an One-Touch Ultra 2. I have been using the same one for over 13 years now. It stopped working as I wrote this chapter. By around September 2007 things had stabilised. My fasting reading on the 16th of September was 109. But to tell you the truth, I never had the opportunity to internalise and understand what type 2 diabetes really is. I was doing a full time job in an ad agency and it left me barely enough time to sleep. **Let me also point out that in 2007 I was never advised to do an HbA1c and neither did anybody warn me of the complications that an unmanaged and uncontrolled diabetes could lead to.**

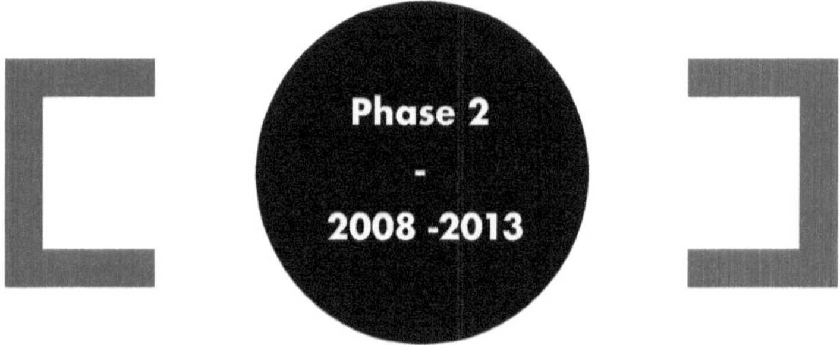

You will be shocked to know that I did not do much about getting my sugar levels under control in these 5 years. I left the ad agency job and moved to the corporate side hoping that there would be a better work-life balance. I was not able to achieve that due to my own conditioning. I liked working late and if I finished work at a reasonable hour then there would be some self-created social engagement to attend. I didn't like coming home early. This vicious cycle continued for 5 long years and I will not be wrong if I say that I probably averaged an a1c of 10 during all those 5 years. I have no idea about the intensity of damage that may have caused my body. I was still with my family doctor then and in 2013 my a1c report actually showed a 10 on it. By this time, while I was still a novice with respect to my knowledge on type 2 diabetes, I was aware of the fact that a 10 is bad. The report descriptions said it. For the first time in my life

I was scared. During this period I did start to realise the ill effects of a badly managed diabetes. I had started hearing about very young people being on dialysis, relatively younger people dying of a heart attack or a stroke and type 2 diabetics being put on insulin.

I think the first time I ever did an HbA1c was in 2013. With a double digit number on the test report I finally decided to quit working full time. I had still not gained enough knowledge to understand that maybe I should move away from my family doctor and see a specialist. I spent the year 2014 trying to lose weight and change my eating habits. This was also the time that I did the 14-day food experiment that I have outlined in chapter 9. But I was still not in the habit of doing my quarterly HbA1cs and hence I could never quantify my progress. I don't think I did a great job of putting all that knowledge into practice and my HbA1c in April 2015 (below) is testimony to that fact.

In 2015 an ex-colleague of mine recommended a very senior diabetologist to me. He is attached to one of the best diabetes-care hospitals in Mumbai and also runs a private practice. I decided to see him at his private clinic.

Here is how I progressed:

Month / Year	HbA1c
April 2015	9.8
Dec 2015	6.4
March 2016	6.0
June 2016	5.3

The experience

- For the first time after becoming a diabetic, I experienced the joy of a brilliant HbA1c.
- I had seriously started working on my food and exercise.
- I started getting treated for hypertension too and I am glad that we did not miss it.
- Things were going fine and my blood sugar levels were really under control.

Despite things going well with this doctor, I was personally very dissatisfied with him due to his very clinical approach. He lacked empathy and this was hampering my interactions with him. In hindsight, I can point to many things he could have done differently. But that may not be the right approach to take in this very positive book.

Finally I bid a goodbye to the 2nd doctor in my diabetes lifecycle. I haven't seen him after the 27th of June 2016.

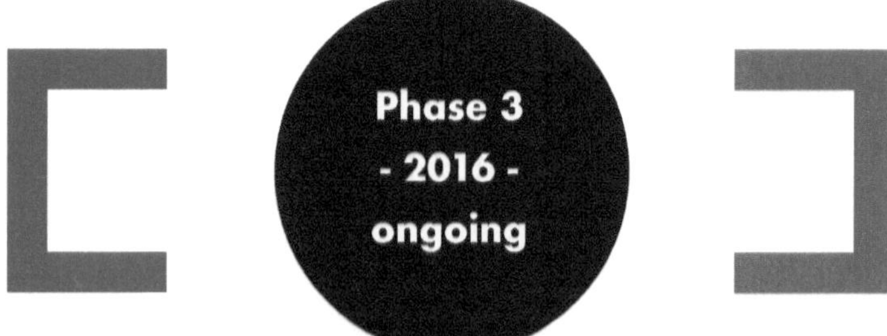

My 3rd doctor is also a specialist. She put me on Glycomet-SR, a slow release metformin. For 4 years now, barring a few changes in doses and timing of the medications, we have been at a status quo until the last quarter of 2020. Here are my readings:

Month / Year	HbA1c
Dec 2016	6.0
Mar 2017	5.9
May 2017	6.3
Aug 2017	5.2
Nov 2017	5.9
Mar 2018	6.2
June 2018	6.3
Sept 2018	6.6
Dec 2018	6.2
April 2019	6.2
July 2019	6.2
Oct 2019	5.9

I missed testing in December 2019 as I had undergone cataract surgeries for both my eyes in November 2019. Was it a diabetic cataract or not, I am not sure. But it was very premature for sure.

Post that in March 2020 the covid 19 pandemic hit the world and the lockdowns began. Here you should recall chapter 5 where I have described the positive effects of intermittent walking and an HbA1c of 5.8 in October 2020. I also realised that this form of walking was doing a lot for me in terms of regulating my blood sugar levels to the extent that I started experiencing hypoglycemia and headaches. This led to a virtual appointment with my doctor and reduction in dosages of Glycomet-SR from 1350mg per day to 1000mg per day. But then my reading in December 2020 increased to a 6.4. What you need to note here is that I didn't walk in that quarter to see the effect of the changed dosage. Food was a constant.

With this on the report my doctor added a small dose of a medicine that takes care of post meal hyperglycemia. I have to now understand the effect of a slow release biguanide + this new medicine on my blood sugar levels. I have been observing that my fasting and postprandial readings after breakfast and lunch are in-range. I am currently working on getting my postprandial readings post dinner right. That is what this quarter (January - March 2021), as I continue writing this chapter, is about.

Trust me. It is a good problem to solve, a good transition to undergo.

This has been my diabetic life so far. I am sure you don't have detailed notes like I do. You should. It is extremely important to keep track of the details of your diabetic life. **Your medicines** and what they do for you. **Your HbA1cs** and how have they moved quarter to quarter. **Your food habits** and how have you evolved them to suit a certain phase of your life and **your exercise** routine.

This
is what I
mean by
transitions and
transformations.

THE ART OF SOCIAL UNDIPLOMACY...

12 ▶ **...learning to say no will be your biggest asset**

This is the final chapter of this book. In the last eleven chapters we learnt about:

- The 8 reasons for hyperglycemia
- The complications of an unmanaged diabetes
- Redefining food and exercise and using them as strategic tools
- Medications, diagnostics and interpretations thereof
- Your relationship with your doctor
- Glycaemic control across your diabetes life-cycle
- And the ultimate short-cut to diabetes management

I hope that these eleven chapters were new and insightful. I hope that each one of them has armed you with enough facts & figures and tricks & tools to help you go about your diabetes management in the most optimal manner. This chapter is qualitative in nature. A bit like chapter 7, wherein we discussed the relationship you have with your doctor and how to improve it. This chapter is about your relationship with your world. There are multiple stakeholders in this world and there are a certain set rules that define the dynamics and interactions you have with them. There is a certain level of conditioning and accordingly a certain level of expectation as far as your societal behaviour goes. This chapter is about the need for you to shake-up and change those rules to benefit you. I have deliberately kept this chapter as the last one as the success of your diabetes management depends on this the most. This is something that I would like to leave you with. Here it is.

When you become diabetic at a relatively younger age, you need to be very careful about your life henceforth. The reason is simple - there is that much more time for the diabetes-related complications to set in. Neuropathy, retinopathy and nephropathy are not far away if you are not able to maintain healthy blood sugar levels reasonably consistently.

> **For being able to do this effectively, you have to not only control and condition your own self well, but also those around you. This may seem daunting at first. But when your survival instinct kicks in, nothing is impossible. Let me emphasise my point through a real story, a story of a type 2 diabetic, who is a kind, benign person, someone who finds it very difficult to say 'no' to people around her and hence today is experiencing the not-so-pleasant consequences of sustained hyperglycemia.**

I have known this lady for over 7 years now. She is probably in her mid-50s and has been a diabetic for over 20 years. Retinopathy has set in 10 years back and her glycaemic control has not been better than a 7 ever on the HbA1c scale. In fact it has touched double digits quite a few times. I hope you appreciate that a 10 on the HbA1c chart corresponds to a dangerous average blood sugar level of 240. Her ophthalmologist has warned her about going blind and she has already undergone a couple of rounds of laser corrections in her eye. She says that she has tried every possible way to get her blood sugar levels under control. Things seem to work fine for a short period of time, but then fall off the track very soon.

I met her in late 2019 and she was in this 'I have lost the battle' mode and announced yet again to me that her blood sugar levels were uncontrollable and had hit a new high of an HbA1c of beyond 10. I tried to talk to her and understand the reasons. Being a diabetic myself, I try to convert every interaction of this nature into learning for myself. Here is the much hidden but a very significant piece of learning.

I had suspected that a singular event (a hospitalisation, the death of a close family member or something severe in nature) may have affected her emotionally and must have been responsible for this dangerous consequence. But as she kept talking to me, I realised that her reasons, to say the least, were 'silly and manageable'. The following were her reasons for her complete lack of control:

- Diwali
- A niece's wedding
- Her daughter visited
- A family member celebrated a restaurant opening
- There were multiple functions and invitations from close and extended family members and friends
- That left no time to exercise
- The weather got colder
- And to top it all - the perennial, omnipresent work-stress

In India, occasions are in abundance. There are no dearth of events, right from childbirth to death. The 7th month of pregnancy, childbirth, child naming ceremonies, thread ceremonies, mundan ceremonies, birthdays, engagements, weddings, the husband completing 80 years of age, and death itself. Unfortunately food (the not-so-healthy variety) is an integral part of each one of these occasions.

In India, we also have a series of festivals month after month. Again each one of them converges into the 'final act of eating' with food playing a dominant role in every celebration. If nothing else, you will suddenly realise that it is a colleague's birthday, a wedding anniversary or your manager's promotion party. Lame, isn't it?

Where will all this end and how much will you eat?
According to me diabetics need to adopt and champion the nuanced art of being 'socially undiplomatic' or 'contextually rude'. You have to refuse to be emotionally blackmailed by a colleague, a neighbour, a friend or a family member. You have to train yourself to tell those people off who constantly tell you that a piece of cake or a sweet will not hurt. Trust me it will.

No wedding, no childbirth, no diwali and no promotion will lose its sheen just because you have decided to take care of yourself.

All these people may feel bad or hurt initially. It doesn't matter. It is your presence that matters, not what you eat. Get them to understand that. They will learn just as we ourselves did. As survivors, as diabetic warriors it is our duty to educate and sensitise the world around us to our special needs and eventually get them to adhere and in fact appreciate and encourage us for what we are trying to achieve. Being able to say 'no' can become your biggest asset as a diabetic.

> **The first eleven chapters of this book help you in 'developing your diabetes quotient'. Developing the art of 'social undiplomacy' will further help you accelerate and optimise your diabetes management process.**

But this will squarely remain a function of how obsessive and compulsive you get about achieving tight glycaemic control. According to me, better sooner than later. Godspeed.

CHA
PTER
EXER
CISE

CHAPTER EXERCISE

Make a list of all your personal and professional obligations. Rate them on a scale of 1 to 10. 1 being least important and 10 most important. Attend only those that you rate > 8. The rest will eat into your 'me' time and work towards upsetting your HbA1c goal.

NOTES

Sr. No.	Professional Obligations	Need to attend on a scale of 1 - 10	Personal Obligations	Need to attend on a scale of 1 - 10
1				
2				
3				

SOURCES IN NO PARTICULAR ORDER ARE:

https://diabetes.diabetesjournals.org/content/57/7/
1768.figures-onlyl

https://www.ncbi.nlm.nih.gov/pmc/articles/
PMC2661582/

https://www.cornerstones4care.com/staying-on-track/
important-things-to-know/the-diabetes-puzzle.html

https://www.webmd.com/diabetes/guide/types-of-
diabetes-mellitus

http://www.diabetesforecast.org/2015/sep-oct/type-2-
diabetes-progression.html

https://www.webmd.com/diabetes/dawn-phenomenon-
or-somogyi-effect

https://www.diabetes.co.uk/what-is-hba1c.html

https://www.ncbi.nlm.nih.gov/pmc/articles/
PMC3912281/

https://www.ncbi.nlm.nih.gov/pmc/articles/PMC4994556/

https://diatribe.org/

https://www.verywellhealth.com/the-doctor-patient-
relationship-188050

https://www.healthlinkbc.ca/health-topics/uq1193abc

www.ingramcontent.com/pod-product-compliance
Lightning Source LLC
Chambersburg PA
CBHW031407250726
48656CB00002B/569